START BEFORE YOU'RE READY

THE POWER OF TAKING ACTION

KELLY YOUNG W/ EMILY STAPLETON

To my BOOTCAMP community:

Whether you've been with me for the past 16 years or joined for just one workout, you are a Bootcamper. Magic happens when we come together to get better. It's got to mean something to you, and your showing up sure means something to me. I love you guys.

To the KBC Dream Team:

Thank you for the work that you've done to make yourself better so you can serve others so beautifully and powerfully. The work we are doing is important, and I couldn't do it without you.

To my dear friend Beth:

We both learned the hard way to start before you're ready, even though you like to always be ready.

To my beloved family:

Andrew, my husband, teammate, and reluctant Bootcamper;

My children: Dalton, Brandon, Cameron, and Lindsay (who would never let me hear the end of it if I didn't mention our Bull Mastiff Reggie);

You have inspired me to be the best version of myself. Thank you for the sacrifices you've made over the years, allowing me to pursue my passion and do what I love. Being your wife and mom will always be my favorite role.

To my dreamer Mom - this is my song on the radio.

To my "it doesn't matter what you do, just be the best at it"
Dad - I will never stop trying because of you.

To my stepmom, Sheila - thank you for teaching me
what family first really means

My siblings who had a huge impact on who I am today

Shanon, the nurturing giver and leader

Kendall, the resilient overcomer

Marc, the keen observer and storyteller

Chris, the dedicated leader carrying on our family's business

Brooke, the tenacious entrepreneur with a heart for community

To my late cousin Brett:

You gave me something very powerful. I'm not sure why you chose
me, but I want you to know I never took your gift for granted.

Table of Contents

Preface

The winter scenery rushed by as I stared out the window. The back seat was cozy, but I was restless. My thoughts flip-flopped between childhood memories and feelings of missing my own children.

It was January 2008, and I sat alone in the back of my Aunt Maureen and Uncle Jim's car. I was on the way home from my dad's funeral. We were driving from Niskayuna, New York, my childhood hometown, to Chantilly, Virginia, back to the current home I shared with my husband and my four kids.

My beloved father, who had always been my pillar of stability, was gone. He was larger than life. Anyone lucky enough to be in his circle would claim they never met anyone like him. He would wear what was comfortable, say what he felt, and do what he wanted. His vast presence was powerful, authentic, and raw. He did it all, and he did it his way.

My father's name was Larry Spraragen, a name I was proud to be connected to. He had established himself as a respected business owner and community member. He raised six kids with his wife Sheila, my stepmom. He exuded an unwavering air of control, showing little patience for actions that deviated from his standards. His demeanor was polarizing as some perceived him as arrogant and unfriendly.

Despite being opposed to his strictness and rules while growing up, I held his viewpoints in high regard. I trusted his opinion on anything.

Even in adulthood, my father remained a reliable source of strength and support. I often considered how he'd react in various situations, knowing his penchant for pushing people to their best. Yet his sternness led me to dedicate much of my life to seeking his approval and striving to make him proud. Without him, I felt lost.

The funeral took place at Proctors Theater, where numerous individuals, including employees, family members, and friends, stood up to speak. What resonated throughout all their words was his tenacity, goodness to people, generosity, the respect he earned for his business acumen, and the deep affection he held in the hearts of many. There were jokes about his tough exterior and high expectations, but the people who knew him best admired his authenticity and genuineness.

My husband had taken our four kids back home, leaving me with my extended family. Though Maureen and Jim aren't blood relatives, I've always had a special relationship with them. Maureen, my stepmom's sister, lived with us when we were kids when Jim was stationed overseas. While I was missing my own kids and husband, I cherished this time to ride home from the funeral with Maureen and Jim.

Sitting in the back of the car on the ride home, I couldn't recall the last time I'd been in the back seat. I was used to being the mom driving a minivan or SUV. Despite feeling numb, I tried to keep things lighthearted and asked, "Can we get some ice cream?" It was as if I were playing the role of a child in the back seat. My memories of car trips with my dad were very different. He would declare from the departure that we would not be stopping and under no circumstances would there be any kind of food in the car. He was vehemently opposed to messes and stickiness, and with six kids, that meant strict rules and no stopping.

During that seemingly endless seven-hour car ride, I was just stuck in my seat, lost in my sadness, staring out the window. On top of all that heaviness, I couldn't shake this weird feeling that I was supposed to be doing something, like I was being called or pulled in somehow.

Before this moment, I wasn't looking for something to do. I was completely content with my life. I was ambitious and motivated throughout my life. I had a graduate degree and a professional career in worksite health promotion for the Department of Defense. I also served as the director of a community health promotion program at Inova Hospital System. My last full-time role was a leadership position at a commercial fitness center in Richmond, Virginia. Once my third son was born and we relocated to Northern Virginia, I found my greatest joy in focusing all my energy and ambition on my family. Being a mom was the best job yet.

This is who I was at the time. I was the mom. That was my primary role. I taught fitness classes part time. Instructing classes allowed me to use my creativity and a strong desire to unite people while still spending plenty of time with my family.

I taught at several local gyms, allowing me to bring my kids to the designated kid zones. My daughter Lindsay was six months old. My sons, six-year-old Dalton, five-year-old Brandon, and three-year-old Cameron, were in elementary school and preschool. I genuinely cherished being a stay-at-home mom. There was nothing about it I didn't love. My husband had a demanding job, and my contribution was managing everything else to make his life less stressful. I had meaningful friendships. The kids had playgroups. We lived in a great neighborhood. The point is, I wasn't looking for anything. I did not feel unfulfilled in any way. I loved everything about my life.

On top of all that, group fitness was my happy place. I would teach, and people would appreciate my class and appreciate me. My life as a mom and my work teaching group fitness worked together so seamlessly. The perfect illustration of that is my memory of Wednesday nights. It was Italian night at home, and the night I taught evening fitness classes at a local gym. I made dinner before I left, got my kids to the kids' zone, and taught class, which ended just as my husband was getting home from work, and then we'd have a family dinner. I remember my hands smelling like garlic the whole time I was teaching. It was part of the routine, and it felt good. It felt right.

January 11, 2008, was a typical chaotic morning, juggling getting my eldest son ready for the bus stop while simultaneously managing my two younger boys. Amid this hustle, a sudden phone call informed me of my father's passing. I dropped to my knees and let out a scream, still in a state of disbelief. Through my tears, I managed to convey to my husband that he needed to take charge and get the kids ready to leave.

Although my dad had unexplained medical symptoms that we knew were neurological, his death was completely unexpected. He was supposed to board a plane to Aruba, his favorite winter getaway, the morning he died. My father was such a powerful presence. I had never imagined my life without him.

As I returned from the funeral to my roles as "mom" and "fitness instructor," I knew a seed had been planted. I didn't know what to do next, so I returned to the life I loved. I returned to caring for my kids, supporting my husband, and bringing people together to exercise.

The moment I first felt the whisper to start and grow a fitness community can be pinpointed to that cold January day in 2008 in the back seat of a car on the way home from my dad's funeral. I was seeking a way to channel my grief into something positive, to create meaning from my sadness and honor the strength of my father.

The answer to that calling can be traced to a single workout, which you'll learn about in Chapter 1. But I didn't become this person or fulfill this calling instantly. The ability to bring people together and the desire to help others was already inside me. I have always genuinely loved others and wanted the best for them, but now, my mission was magnified and with purpose. Hundreds (maybe thousands) of life experiences influenced my passion, purpose, and mission.

Introduction

I believe in you. I believe you can achieve your goals and dreams. You might be thinking that I don't even know you—that your dream is too big or your goal too far away. How could I possibly believe in your success?

You might not even believe in yourself. That's OK. I'll believe in you first. You'll catch up. Let's take this journey together.

Why are you here? What are you looking for in this book? Did you pick this book up because you want to change the voice in your head? Do you want to make your life better in some way? I believe we can do that together.

This book is a journey from where you are now to where you should be. I'll share my heart and soul with you. You'll see how, throughout my life, I've taken steps to get from one place to another. If I can do it, so can you.

Let's start with where you are right now. I don't necessarily mean where you are physically, but maybe. But maybe it's where you are in your career, your fitness journey, or your relationship journey—any part of your life that you want to improve.

Then, let's think about where you want to go, where you're supposed to be. Again, maybe where you physically want to go/ where you want to be spiritually. In your career. In your fitness journey. You get the idea.

I know you can get from where you are now to where you should be. But here's what you need to know. There might be many, many steps along the way. Some steps can be challenging and take a long time when working toward a goal. These difficult phases will test your resolve and commitment. However, overcoming them builds resilience and understanding, proving that patience and persistence are key to significant accomplishments. I'll help you take a single step in the right direction—then another, and then another.

Throughout my life, I've experienced life's highest highs and lowest lows. My experiences during childhood, the jobs I've had, my role as a daughter, wife, and mother, and my work in the fitness industry have all shaped who I am today and who I'm becoming. I know you're on a journey that makes you who you are. I also know that we make daily choices that contribute to our experiences. Things don't just happen to us. Experiences shape us, but we also shape our own experiences.

I believe in the power of our paths already paved for us, awaiting our discovery if we tune into the whispers of the universe guiding us toward our true calling and authenticity. Throughout my life, I've encountered numerous challenges. Yet I've shown resilience and strength, virtues instilled in me by three loving parents.

As founder and owner of Kelly's Bootcamp and Inergy, I've worked with hundreds of clients to help them reach their fitness goals. I've learned a lot along the way. Maybe the most important thing I've learned is that it's not just about fitness—but fitness matters.

This isn't a book about becoming physically fit. I won't be giving you a step-by-step guide to getting fit. However, my own life and the experiences of my bootcampers have taught me that fitness is a catalyst for everything else. Fitness teaches us discipline, perseverance, and the importance of self-care—essential qualities for success in every aspect of life.

Fitness teaches us how to move in the right direction. Fitness gives us something concrete to work toward.

When you care enough about your physical body to keep it healthy, everything else will follow. Likewise, if you care enough about everything else (career, relationships, spirituality), you'll care for your physical body.

So wherever you are and wherever you want to go, we'll use fitness to get you there. Working toward your improved physical fitness can get you there. Learning from the stories of my fitness community can propel you in the right direction. Even reliving experiences from your past can move you closer to where you want to be today.

Each chapter of this book contains personal stories and encouragement to help you take a step in the right direction. The stories are mine, but they're also ours. Every person who's ever participated in a workout or event that I've led, been a member of the Kelly's Bootcamp (KBC) community, or been a team member or coach is our story.

In each chapter, I've shared stories from members of our community in their own words. We interviewed each of them, allowing them to introduce themselves and their involvement in KBC. I hope that it gives you some insight into our culture.

I hope, page by page, you'll start to understand where I come from, where I am, and where I'm going.

The words of encouragement in each chapter are short phrases I've used hundreds of times in my fitness business. They're simple, tried and true words that will help you not overthink but instead act.

Sometimes, all we need is an encouraging word or phrase to get us moving toward our goal. Sometimes, by sharing our own experiences with each other, we can motivate a fellow human to reach his or her goal. This book is my opportunity to share my experiences with you and provide some words of encouragement so you can take the next step. And the next. And the next.

The chapters that follow are divided into three parts.

- **My Stories.** I hope that by reading stories from my life, you'll see your own story in a new light. In addition to sharing my personal experiences, I'll impart some words of wisdom in the form of mantras commonly used in my fitness community, Kelly's Bootcamp (KBC).

- **Stories from the Community.** By reading about the passion and transformations of members of the KBC community, I'm certain you'll feel inspired.

- **Kelly's Take.** I've shared my own take on the stories shared by community members.

So let's get started.

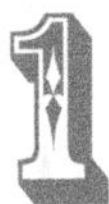

I Already Believe in You

Nearly a year after my dad's death, after the seed was planted on that car ride home, my extended family and I decided to run a half marathon in honor of my dad. None of us were runners, but the race was on his birthday. It was in Las Vegas at night. It was a way for us to put our energy into something positive and honor my dad. We had been following a six-month training plan that my Uncle Jim put together.

We called our team Scuba Squad. Scuba was a nickname my dad first earned when my high school friend dropped her sunglasses into Lake George, and my dad dove in and miraculously came back up with them. That's the kind of thing you could expect from my dad.

While several of us exercised regularly, we weren't runners. But we were doing this. I loved the idea of doing it as a group and being on a team again. There were twenty-seven of us, family and friends, who ran the race together.

Then Uncle Jim suggested that to add more purpose to the race, we should do a fundraiser to support the neurological disease that shortened my dad's life to sixty-one. I wasn't good at asking people for money. I remember some of my family members giving suggestions on how to raise money. I thought, "I'm not doing that." I just hated asking people for money. The only idea I could come up with to raise funds was to host a workout. It was what I knew.

I now realize that the training plan and communications that my uncle sent for our weekly training were also part of the seed that was being planted. Being on a team was my happy place during a tough chapter of my life. Training for something meaningful with a group of people I cared about was **More Than Just a Workout**.

Here's an excerpt from one of Uncle Jim's many communications.

"We should add a greater sense of purpose to this event. Collectively, we should designate a fundraising goal (with planned events like happy hours) to raise money for something of significance to Larry. Sheila and family should decide on the charity we'll support. We don't have to do this, but I think it'll make the whole weekend that much more meaningful.

My whole reason for doing this race was to honor Larry and celebrate his birthday. He was without a doubt my greatest Team in Training and Leukemia and Lymphoma Society supporter over the years. He was such a generous benefactor to so many charities and organizations; I think he would be proud to know that we're doing this as a family for a greater purpose than just crossing the finish line.

Running and coaching have been such an important part of my life for so many years; I'm thrilled that I'll be able to share this experience with the family. I always tell my athletes to respect the distance, not fear it—13.1 miles is not an easy thing, but I know that each and every one of you can do it. We'll have finishers well under two hours, and we'll have folks over three hours. The most important thing is that we'll be there to support each other and celebrate a collective accomplishment."

The weekend before the race was Thanksgiving, and my stepmom, Sheila, and some of my siblings were coming from New York to stay with me in Virginia. It was the first Thanksgiving without my dad. I decided to host an outdoor workout to bring people together, burn off some Thanksgiving calories, and raise money for Team Scuba. I called my fundraiser Black Friday Bootcamp.

At first, I didn't really think anyone would come. I was checking a box. I was not super excited about it. Uncle Jim wanted us to raise money, so I was doing it. I just wanted to bring people together. It's the day after Thanksgiving. Everyone will want to move their bodies. But honestly, I didn't have any expectations.

I made a flyer. And then, one night, after I taught fitness class, I got up the nerve to tell my students about it. I remember holding the paper in my hand and reading it. My hand was shaking. It made me so uncomfortable to ask people to do something and to ask for money on top of that.

The next time I taught, I was walking down the hall and heard someone yell my name. A woman who had taken my classes handed me a check and said, "Hey, I'd love to go to your event, but I'm not available that day. But I want to contribute." I remember looking down at the check and seeing the names Virginia and Chris Katz, and I was just so blown away that she was so thoughtful and generous to track me down and write out the check. It was symbolic to me. This one person helped me believe that people would come to the workout. And then people did come. In addition to my own extended family, we had about thirty neighbors and friends show up at our community tennis courts for a bootcamp-style station workout.

I cherished witnessing families engage in a workout together. The air was crisp, but the sun was shining, casting a golden glow. My dad loved the sun. It felt like he was with us. My dad and I used to play basketball and tennis together. The Black Friday Bootcamp took place on the tennis courts of my neighborhood clubhouse. My kids, stepmom, aunts, uncles, cousins, and younger siblings were there. Everyone was happy. It was a simple format. I didn't overthink it, and I wanted people to feel successful. I felt so connected to the group; our time together during that workout session was magical.

It was **More Than Just a Workout**. Sometimes, feelings and emotions go beyond the normal response to working out, beyond "I'm sweating, I'm working my muscles." When you come together with other people in a shared space, doing similar things, no matter where you're coming from, no matter what else is going on in your life, there's something that's created: a group feeling of accomplishment, a connection that's created when people are getting uncomfortable with the physical part of the workout. Then maybe there's somebody next to you who cheers for you or says something encouraging. It's just a really special energy. It's simple but really powerful, and there's always something deeper going on. It reminds us that if we show up strong here, we can show up strong in other places.

Despite this being the first holiday season without my father, I could feel joy and connection. The positive energy in the air was palpable. I was proud of the work I had done to facilitate the workout, especially knowing that people were having fun and bettering themselves at the same time. I know my dad would have teased me about a tennis court workout and had something funny to say, but I also know he would be proud.

As soon as I finished the Black Friday Bootcamp, I knew this was it. This was the calling, the thing I was supposed to do. It was very significant. There was no doubt. I knew with 100% certainty that I was supposed to be doing this. The whisper from the back of the car was starting to make sense.

I never looked back. That single workout led to another bootcamp and then to another. Those thirty people led to another person, and then another, and then to more people.

I didn't have any expectations, and I didn't have an official business plan. I'm a doer, so right away, I just thought, *I'm going to do this*. I picked March 1 to start. And from there, everything happened organically. Kelly's Bootcamp (KBC) was born.

I remained focused on my newfound desire to create a fitness community. I felt aligned with what I was supposed to be doing and let things happen naturally. I wasn't in a hurry. I just followed my calling and my passion.

I hosted a single workout on Black Friday. Then, four months later, I started hosting Saturday morning workouts outdoors. It was originally supposed to be one class, but I added a second because of the demand and because couples with small children needed to come at different times so that one parent could manage the kids. I just kept moving forward to meet people's needs. People would ask for something, and then I would figure out how to offer it. I added more weekday classes and an indoor facility eight years later.

Eventually, that Black Friday Bootcamp led to an LLC, a wrapped cargo van filled with fitness equipment, a team of talented and accredited instructors, a dedicated community of over 400 active clients, a beautiful indoor training studio, and a thriving business that serves a community beyond anything I could have planned or imagined.

I took a risky path with minimal direction. There was no business plan, niche market, or sense of where I wanted to go. I had an overall mission to promote health and prevent sickness. My passion and purpose guided every move.

This calling did not come out of nowhere. In the back seat of a car after my dad's funeral, it felt like a whisper. However, my desire to assist individuals in prioritizing good health started years ago.

One of the most important things I want you to get from this book is the ability to tap into the whispers that you hear. The whispers changed my life; they seemed random, but my path was there. I just needed to be open to and willing to do the work. I've learned that **If You Want Something Bad Enough, You'll Find a Way to Make It Happen**. You may need to let go of other things you thought you wanted. Some things may feel like a waste.

My waste and my redos were my pivotal moments. I didn't know it then, but as I look back, I see how every little thing added up and brought me somewhere wonderful and exactly where I was supposed to be. I will share more details later, but there was a pivotal moment when I knew I needed to take my life in a different direction from my current college curriculum.

This book explores where you've been and where you want to go and encourages you to pay attention to the signs and whispers you see and hear along the way. Although I didn't have a clear plan for what would eventually become my fitness business, I knew I had a mission. And I knew what my purpose was. I believed in myself.

I Already Believe in You. I believe you can achieve your goals and dreams.

You might be thinking that you don't even believe in yourself. That's OK. I'll believe in you first. Let's take this journey together.

More Than Just a Workout

Feelings and emotions go beyond the normal response to working out, beyond, "I'm sweating. I'm working my muscles." It's when you come together in a shared space, doing similar things. No matter where you're coming from or what else is going on in your life, there's something that's created—a group feeling of accomplishment, a connection created when people are getting uncomfortable with the physical part of the workout. There's something deeper going on. It reminds us that if we show up strong here, we can show up strong in other places.

If You Want Something Badly Enough, You Will Find a Way to Make It Happen

If you really value something, you'll find a way to make it happen. If it's not happening, it's probably not really that important to you. That's where being more strategic with your time becomes essential. If you really want it badly enough, you'll find time and energy to make it happen. If not, maybe you should take it off your list.

I Already Believe in You

Sometimes, you need someone else to believe in you before you even believe in yourself. That belief from someone else can and will eventually help you believe in yourself.

Debbie's Story

In the spring of 2009, my neighbor and close friend, Cindy, informed me that she had started attending a bootcamp. While she was a runner,

I didn't consider myself an athlete. Cindy encouraged me to join in with her, but she suggested that I should first have a one-on-one meeting with Kelly, the instructor.

I recently visited the doctor and weighed in at 225 pounds. I was experiencing difficulty carrying out daily activities and caring for my children. Climbing stairs left me out of breath, and I was feeling very unhealthy. My cholesterol levels were high, and the doctor suggested medication unless I made changes to my diet and exercise routine. I scheduled an appointment with Kelly at her house.

She was encouraging and pretty straightforward. Kelly was very clear: "I don't want anybody that's wishy-washy. I don't want anybody that's halfway. If you're here, you're doing this. Let's go!" We went through several exercises: squats, sit-ups, and pushups to see what I could do. It was quick because I couldn't do very many.

I can't say that Kelly was warm and fuzzy, but I was drawn to her. She showed up to the workouts, no matter what. That was her mindset: cold, rain, sleet, snow, 100 degrees. No matter what, she had that truck, equipment, and a little envelope in the front seat where you threw in five bucks. From the beginning, it was always a labor of love and a passion for helping people improve. I believed back then that she wanted me to get better. She wanted me to get stronger. She wanted me to feel good.

Initially, my goal was weight loss and looking great in an outfit. But it has become so much more than that. I noticed in Kelly that she believed in me from the beginning. I didn't believe in myself. I just showed up. And the more she offered me, the more I would attend. I started one day a week, and I went every time. And then she said, "I will provide this another day and time." I was like, "I'll be there." And then it became five days a week, then six. I couldn't get enough of it.

I grew up in the KBC community. I have experienced tremendous loss in my life. I've lost six people, including Cindy Comeau (my dear friend who got me started with KBC), to a brain tumor. I have a daughter who has struggled with mental health and substance abuse for the past six years. This community has saved me. Being a part of KBC means having somewhere to go where I know that people love me and want me to be there and they miss me when I'm not there. I miss them when I'm not there.

It has unearthed deep feelings about all those people I've lost. But it also reminds me of how vital this community is to me.

One significant moment occurred during a run club class with Kelly when I doubted my capabilities. Her response, emphasizing the importance of maintaining a growth mindset, resonated deeply with me. According to Kelly, there's always room for improvement if one is willing to put in the effort.

I teach educators for Fairfax County government, and we talk about growth mindset. I have since taken courses built around Carol Dweck. Dweck is a renowned psychologist known for her groundbreaking research on mindset. She introduced the concepts of "fixed mindset" and "growth mindset," explaining how individuals' beliefs about their abilities significantly impact their learning and success. Dweck's work demonstrates that those with a growth mindset, who believe abilities can be developed through effort and learning, are more likely to overcome challenges and achieve higher success levels than those with a fixed mindset, who see abilities as static and unchangeable. Kelly talked about getting out of your fixed mindset and remembering that there were always growth opportunities ten years ago. Kelly helps us believe there's always room for improvement if you keep showing up and working at it. It's always there for the taking. It's always ready for you.

I'm known for being social and welcoming at KBC because I want to love people who are there the way that I feel loved when I'm there. So I will show up that way because it matters. I want people to come there, feel welcome, and want to come back. Nobody asked me to do that, but that's my thing. That's where I feel the strongest and the most useful. That's really where my heart is. How can I serve the community that has done so much for me?

Brene Brown's work on belonging explores the deep human need to feel connected and accepted. Brown emphasizes that true belonging requires individuals to be authentic and embrace their vulnerabilities rather than conforming to fit in.

She talks about fitting in and belonging. She shares that the opposite of fitting in is belonging because fitting in is trying to make yourself into something to be a part of the group. Belonging is when you're already with people who accept you for exactly who you are. That's what I want to be. That's who I want to show up as. That's how I feel when I'm there. It starts with Kelly; I've seen her passionately showing up for people time after time.

I'm forever sharing the tips, tricks, and things I've learned from KBC with my friends and family. My biggest advice to anyone trying to change is to ask for what you need. Three years ago, after many years of losing weight and gaining it back, I asked Kelly if I could get on the Inbody composition scale at the beginning of every month and share my results to stay accountable. An InBody composition scale is a device that measures body composition using Bioelectrical Impedance Analysis (BIA). It sends low-level electrical currents through the body to assess the amount of body fat, muscle mass, and water distribution. The results provide a detailed breakdown of these components, helping users understand their overall body composition and track changes over time.

I had great success, and others asked to do it too. In response, Kelly created a program called the DW (my initials and nickname). This program invites members to get on the Inbody every month all year long. With that ongoing accountability, I have lost fifty pounds, 14% body fat, and increased my skeletal muscle mass. In the months my numbers are not great, she picks out the positive things and sees the big picture.

In the program's first year, fifty-five individuals enrolled; this year, sixty-five people signed up. It brings tears of joy to my eyes to see that I have been able to be a catalyst for a program that is helping so many people with sustainable changes. Seeing its positive impact on people's lives is personally rewarding and a significant way for me to give back. Furthermore, the fact that some people signed up for the program because of my success adds another layer of accountability for me.

Kelly's Take

You should think of a specific person when you have a product or a program. Debbie has been that person for me. When she started fifteen years ago, she was not serious about exercise or weight loss, but she fell in love with the process of showing up, and from there, anything was possible. Her success and enthusiasm gave me confidence as I was starting. Debbie also had a significant role in KBC's outreach to needy people.

Debbie's gratitude for the community was palpable, and she significantly expanded KBC's reach. Whenever Debbie noticed a community need, she approached me with ideas to address it. When a family in our community experienced a devastating townhouse fire, Debbie suggested we organize a Bootcamp fundraiser to support them. She also facilitated connections between KBC and initiatives like Race for a Cure, rallying our community to support causes like brain tumor research. We've held special workouts in memory of a well-loved breast cancer warrior and organized a dinosaur-themed workout fundraiser for a young boy diagnosed with cancer.

One of the most memorable classes of my life was with Cindy's extended family on the day of her funeral. I remember being so nervous when Debbie asked me to host it, but I have learned that it's always the right thing to do when your heart is in the right place.

Debbie's compassion and actions have profoundly impacted our community, fostering greater connectedness and empathy. I sincerely appreciate how she emphasizes the power of showing up and resilience. It's a principle that resonates deeply with me as I strive to lead by example as an instructor. Debbie's dedication to fitness and helping others become their best version is inspiring. Just as she found success through consistent effort and growth in her fitness journey, the same applies to other areas of her life.

I admire Debbie's acknowledgment of the social aspect of our community, which has undoubtedly played a pivotal role in her success story. By surrounding herself with like-minded, caring, and health-conscious people, Debbie has created a supportive environment where everyone feels welcome. She has a knack for bringing people together and fostering a sense of belonging, which has been instrumental in her journey and the success of others.

Debbie's transformation inspires many, and I am thrilled that friends and family reach out to her for advice. As she mentioned, she signed up as KBC evolved with additional programming, such as nutrition coaching and small groups. She built upon her own success, always willing to invest in herself and learn. Tiny changes over time led to a massive transformation. There was no quick fix or magic pill. Her journey was challenging, emotional, and long. It will never be over, but her likelihood of continued success is high due to how being healthy and fit makes her feel and because she has fallen in love with the process, not just the outcome.

Debbie said something simple but powerful: Find what you need. If someone doesn't have a solution to your problem, create one. One of the things that I am most proud of as a small business owner is the connection I can have with our members. They are constantly giving us feedback and expressing what they want and need. The DW is a year-long accountability program that involves a monthly Inbody check-in. The Inbody is a powerful tool for sustainable body composition change because the goal is to keep or increase muscle, which makes you more metabolic and more likely for long-term success.

Debbie did this independently, and when another member asked if she could do it, I knew more people would be interested. 2024 is the third year of the DW (Debbie's fourth), and we have made improvements yearly. We have set expectations for graduation and peer accountability to increase compliance. We made a big deal about those who successfully completed the program because they did something every month for a year. The results don't have to be great, but you have to do it no matter what. It's a compelling program created by an iconic student who cares just as much about helping others as she does about herself.

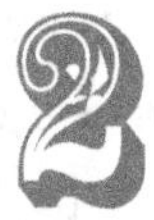

Just Show Up

Everyone has a story. Our unique stories start with influences from early childhood, and they shape the trajectory of our lives. Here's my story as best I can remember it. It begins with the story of my mom and dad.

I was in the lower level garage of the country home my parents had built in Burnt Hills, New York—an eight-year-old girl wearing a pink nightgown with a hippopotamus. I remember how cold the floor felt on my feet and how big and wet the tears felt on my face. My father, usually a figure of strength and authority, stood before me with a bag slung over his shoulder, speaking softly in a tone I had never heard. He reassured me he wasn't leaving me, just my mom.

A mix of determination and sorrow played across his face as he stood there. His once-imposing figure seemed diminished in the dim light, burdened by the weight of his decision. I pleaded with him to stay, unable to comprehend the distinction between him leaving me and leaving my mom. Despite his attempts to comfort me, his words felt feeble as he eventually drove away, leaving me alone on the tear-stained garage floor.

In the days following, my mom struggled to cope. She locked herself in her room, overwhelmed by the situation. This was too much for her to handle, and when things got hard, she escaped to becoming a different person. I knocked on the door to see if she was OK. I remember my dad calling and checking in. I was angry at him, but I also needed to hear his voice.

My brother Kendall, who is just fourteen months older than me, was there too. Kendall had always been my dad's right-hand man. He went everywhere with my dad. They built a barn on our property together, washed the cars, and mowed the lawn. Growing up, Kendall was the golden child to my dad. He was admired for his mechanical skills, hard work ethic, and physical strength. Our parents' divorce and the changes that it brought had a profound effect on my brother Kendall. He struggled with emotional distress and, in seeking relief, resorted to destructive behaviors to cope with his frustrations and anger.

On the other hand, I always wanted to be with my mom. With her long, jet-black hair framing her slender figure, she possessed an enormous smile that would light up the room, although it was not always present due to her struggles with mental illness. Despite this, I wanted to be by her side, especially when she was doing the things she loved, as that's when her happiness shined the brightest.

In the kitchen, she would give me small jobs that had to be performed to her exact specifications. With precision, she instructed me on the exact baking method: First, carefully spoon the flour into the measuring cup, making sure not to pack it down. Then, using the flat side of a knife, level off the flour so it's perfectly even with the rim of the cup.

Other times, she'd spend the night sewing, creating her own patterns. I would often find myself curled up under the large table in her meticulously organized sewing room, surrounded by the comforting hum of the sewing machine and the rhythmic snipping sound as the blades glided through the fibers of the fabric.

I would listen to her play guitar and sing as she drank coffee and smoked Saratoga brand cigarettes, one after the other. My mom's voice had a twangy quality that added authenticity to her storytelling, blending vulnerability with a gritty vocal delivery. Her voice carried a depth of emotion that I would later begin to fear as I knew it usually meant she would have an episode of sickness coming soon.

After my dad left, my mom got sick. I didn't fully understand what that meant. All I knew was that it meant she would go into the hospital (sometimes for a long time), and when she came back out, she would be really happy and want to spend lots of time with me. When my parents were together, my father would get help for Kendall and me when she went into the hospital. Once they were separated, we would live with my dad until she was ready to care for us again.

I later discovered that my mom's first bipolar episode happened before she met my dad when she was just nineteen. Giving birth to a baby she ultimately gave up for adoption deeply affected her, leaving a lasting trauma that manifested in hallucinations and seeing the baby again. The trauma from that experience led to the first of many extended visits to the psychiatric ward. While that difficult situation was the catalyst, bipolar disorder is characterized by chemical imbalances in the brain, and she was predisposed to the disease by other factors. My mother never got sick when she was pregnant with Kendall or me, but her illness undoubtedly placed a heavy burden on my father when we were little.

He had to juggle providing for us while safeguarding her and our family. According to what I've been told, two specific events prompted my father to realize the need to change our family dynamic. One involved her attempting to give me away to a neighbor, while the other was the decision to put our beloved family dog to sleep. These incidents underscored the severity of her illness and the strain it placed on our family.

My parents had a very contentious divorce. Kendall and I were very involved in the proceedings, much more than kids today are. I remember lawyers and doctors asking us lots of questions about my mom, trying to get us to say bad things. I hated my dad for what he was doing to my mom, and I equally resented my mom for putting me in this position. This marked the onset of my guilt and anxiety.

The custody battle continued. My dad fought hard for our well-being, and my mom fought with her heart. We were her babies, and even though she was not capable of caring for us at times, I never doubted how much she loved us. It was not an easy childhood, but we were always provided for and loved. My parents fought for us with every bit of money and power they had. It was a battle that nobody would ever win.

Ultimately, my dad got custody. I was ten years old when my father married Sheila. Sheila also had two children, Shanon (twelve at the time) and Marc (eleven). Kendall and I moved in with a new stepmom, stepsister, stepbrother, and half-brother Chris, and five years later, our half-sister Brooke was born.

With the addition of a stepmom, stepsiblings, and half-siblings, my life has become a mix of blessings and challenges. My stepsister, Shanon, became my closest friend and confidant. Marc, our stepbrother, and Kendall hung out together. My little brother, Chris, was the center of my heart and connected this newly formed family. Chris was adored by all four of his older siblings, and as he got older and started obsessing with He-man figures, we would fight over who was going to buy Chris the newest character. I tread carefully in my interactions with my step-mom Sheila out of respect for my mother's feelings. She seemed really nice and fun, but she was not my mom.

During my parents' divorce, I was in elementary school. I moved schools abruptly when my mom was sick and switched back and forth between Niskayuna and Burnt Hills in fifth grade. Once the custody battle ended and we were with my dad, Kendall and I settled at Niska-yuna.

When we first went to live with my dad and Sheila, I was full of emotion because I was worried about my mom, and I didn't want to leave her. I felt very guilty. There was a time before Kendall and I switched schools when Sheila would drive us to Burnt Hills. Even as a fifth grader, I knew this was a lot for her, and I felt bad about it. Kendall and I were both resistant to switching schools, and as expected, there were lots of questions from other students about why we left and came back, why we couldn't live with our mom, and whether or not we would actually be staying this time.

Despite my worries and sadness, I made many new friends at my new school. I was a good student, and school was vital to me. Even then, I thought I had to **Just Show Up**, so I did. I went to my new school and did my best. I developed strong relationships with friends, teachers, and coaches.

At Burnt Hills, the first school I attended, I was tagged as talented and gifted. It was my favorite thing about school because it felt special. We'd have these cool separate classroom sessions a few times a week with comfortable chairs and a fish tank. We had the opportunity to collaborate and work on group projects. I was totally in my element.

At my new school, Niskayuna, I didn't qualify for the program. It hit me hard because being a good student was a big part of my identity.

With so many other changes happening, this left me feeling vulnerable and insecure. I started doubting my abilities in school, questioning if I really was a good student.

I thought I didn't qualify for the program at Niskayuna because I was no longer as smart as I used to be. Looking back, I now understand that the caliber of students was probably higher at Niskayuna, and the criteria for their program were most likely different. It had nothing to do with my abilities changing. Still, at that time, I decided that I was no longer considered intelligent.

This started a limiting belief I had carried for a long time. It can be hard to overcome once you get a limiting belief in your head. I carried that belief around with me for a long time.

The belief that I wasn't smart didn't stop me from loving school and working very hard to earn good grades. But it became increasingly obvious that I had to work harder than many other kids in that school. School no longer came easy to me.

As you'll learn in future chapters, my early jobs, parenting, and fitness business gave me additional opportunities to Just Show Up and work hard.

At KBC, **Just Show Up** is at the heart of our community culture. It's what I want my members to experience when they come to a workout. I want people to feel like when they walk in the door of Inergy or arrive at the lot, all their worries are gone. Everything is taken care of. I want their workout to be a transformative physical and mental experience. They just need to show up and allow themselves to check out of work stress, family concerns, what's for dinner, put the phone away and let us take care of the rest.

When you show up, it allows you to **Get What You Came For**. When KBC members come to a workout, they're all getting something different out of it. Maybe they're here because they need to hear the message that your best is always good enough. Maybe they're here because they will help the person next to them and know that being here will give that person a better workout. Maybe it is the only hour in the day that is just about them and no one else. Those are things that can happen when you **Just Show Up**. It means don't overthink it. You don't have to be the best. You don't have to know what you're doing. You don't have to understand fitness. You don't even need to know what to expect.

For decades, I've been encouraging my fitness clients to go after their goals and achieve something that feels impossible. If you want something badly enough, you make it happen. With purpose and passion, anything is possible.

Know your why and let it dictate your every move—where there is a why, there is a way.

In the book "Find Your Why," Simon Sinek says, "If we want to feel an undying passion for our work, if we want to feel we are contributing to something bigger than ourselves, we all need to know our *why*."

Defining and knowing your why is the key to living with passion. Usually, our *why* is more significant than ourselves. People will always do more for others than they'll do for themselves. Knowing what your *why* is and who it will impact is an essential step to moving in the right direction.

What is my *why*? I have a story. I believe that my story will help other people. My story doesn't involve any unachievable superstar talents. I **Just Show Up**—always. I always work hard, and I always find a way to get better. My superpower is that I have no superpower. I just keep showing up.

My current *why*, the reason I'm writing this book, is that I want to help other people by sharing my own story. My story of growing up, my story of working hard, my story of parenting, and my story of building a thriving fitness community.

It's a story anyone can learn from and act on. My story is that I have always believed in myself. I was never particularly gifted in any area, but I have always believed I could make it happen. I also believe that I can outwork anyone. I don't have to be the best. I just need to stick with it and keep going when other people get tired. The belief that hard work could and would pay off started when I was just a kid in middle school.

What is your *why*? Your why can change and evolve based on the situation or the season of life. Your *why* might date back to your childhood. Or you might be dreaming up a new *why* right this minute. The important thing is that you define your *why* and then really go for it. Show up. Work hard. Don't stop.

Just Show Up

Start by showing up. Don't overthink it. You don't have to be the best. You don't have to know what you're doing. You don't have to understand fitness. You don't even need to know what to expect.

Get What You Came For

When you show up for a workout or anything else, you can get what you need. Ask yourself, what did I come here for today? What you need can change, and it might be very different from what someone else needs or what you might need tomorrow. It's very fluid and individualized.

Know Your *Why*

Where there's a *why*, there's a way. When you know why you want to do something, you're much more likely to do it. Your *why* can evolve throughout your life. The important thing is to define your right-now *why*. Then let it dictate your every move.

Amy's Story

I started my first job the day I turned fifteen. I was the babysitter in the tiny closet of a room down the hall from the aerobics studio in the main fitness center in my small hometown. Other than routine babysitting jobs and being the oldest of three kids, I had no experience with toddlers, much less babies. Yet here I was, being handed screaming infants while their moms dashed off late to catch an aerobics class. It wasn't glamorous, and the minutes crept by, but I had a job, making my own money ($3.35 an hour), and an unexpected perk: taking all the aerobics classes I wanted.

I quickly moved up to the front desk position as soon as possible and worked there through high school and even a few breaks during college. It was my first exposure to the magic of group fitness, and I remember idolizing the instructors, getting to class early so I could get my spot, and feeling like I was floating on clouds after leaving class.

I was a cheerleader for the University of Virginia football and basketball teams during college, which fed my passion for movement, music, and great people. I stopped and started at different gyms a few times during my twenties and early thirties, but nothing I really fell in love with enough to drive any consistency.

I definitely felt like a piece of me was missing during my early twenties, as I graduated, started working full time, got married, and went to grad school to get a teaching degree. I felt a little lost, and I think part of that was not having a team or community to be a part of. Throughout the following decade and a half, my husband and I grew our family, and I decided to become a stay-at-home mom to our three boys.

Besides lots of walks to try and wear the boys out, I did not do any fitness during this time. My eating was mostly quick convenience foods. I was in survival mode and not focused on my own health and well-being.

I reached a point where my weight was at an all-time high, and ironically enough, I remember being in Moe's eating nachos when I got a Facebook notification that a friend we had just vacationed with posted a picture of me. I remember immediately pulling it up on my phone and being horrified to see myself in a very unflattering bathing suit picture. I immediately untagged myself. I couldn't untag the image from my mind, though. What had happened to me?

In January 2012, I made a New Year's resolution to attend one class per week at the community rec center. My friend had found a Saturday morning cardio dance class, and we attended together. It was so great to be back moving my body, listening to great music, and just having me-time. I kept that class up, eventually added one more, and started eating a little better. Within just six months, I was down ten pounds and feeling a little bit like my old self again. When the instructor I liked at the rec center announced she was moving, I began desperately looking for an alternative.

That month at the beach, I ran into a longtime friend, Brandon Pugh, who noticed I had lost some weight and suggested I come to his bootcamp. I heard the word "bootcamp" and thought of endless pushups and burpees on a park bench with someone screaming at me. And I thought, no, thank you. I'm not a bootcamp person! I like music, rhythm, and fun fitness. I just thought that wasn't for me. Apparently destiny had other plans.

A few months later, I noticed my youngest son's preschool teacher looked very fit and had fantastic energy, so I asked her where she worked out. She said, "Kelly's Bootcamp. You should come. You would love it!"

I found Kelly's information online and emailed her. Knowing me, I had a long email written with background info, asking all about the classes, what I needed to do, asking about pricing, etc. She replied quickly and briefly that she would love for me to come. Just show up! I appreciated not having to go through a whole process, but I was still apprehensive and nervous. While I had worked out in fitness studios, this workout class took place outdoors in the parking lot of a shopping center. It seemed a bit odd. But I did—I showed up in a parking lot with my water bottle and exercise mat. My first memory is of good music. That was a big mental check for me. Then, Kelly and the people who were all so friendly were moving the way I had in those aerobics classes so long ago. I was hooked from the first class.

Within the first three months, I went from attending once or twice a week to probably five days a week, anytime I could get there. My husband supported me, and we often swapped off with the kids in the parking lot. I was becoming different and showing up for myself and my family in new and better ways. It was a gradual transition but one in which I quickly would not recognize that former version of myself on the beach. I was confident again in my physical appearance, which translated into everything I did.

It was very easy to get to know the people in class—many were moms like me. About five or six months in, I missed one of my regular classes, and I remember someone texting me and saying, "Hey, I wanted to make sure you were OK. You weren't in class." I don't even know how she got my number. That has always stuck with me over ten years later. People care if you're not there.

Almost one year after starting KBC, my middle son, Lex, was diagnosed with Type I diabetes. It was devastating and overwhelming, and I became obsessed with learning about nutrition and helping him thrive. Before that, I was not very educated on nutrition, occasionally grabbing a box of frozen taquitos from Costco and heating them for dinner. I was a grab-and-go girl, trying to survive with three young, hungry boys. I had done a little better since starting to work out, but I still had many fast food convenience options and not many whole foods. When Lex had to change how he ate, I knew the whole family would have to transition. I spent the next year and a half educating myself on not just diabetes but everything about nutrition I could learn. I read, took courses, started cooking more, experimenting with foods, and transitioning very slowly how we all ate, and I noticed significant benefits in how we looked and felt.

In December 2014, Kelly approached me about captaining the 2015 Winter Challenge. The Winter Challenge is a body transformation contest Kelly runs yearly, with teams competing in weight loss, body fat loss, and team challenges. I had heard about it the previous two years, but I was unclear about what was involved and was somewhat intimidated by the whole thing. I was flattered, though, that Kelly thought to ask me, and after thinking it over, I texted her that I could co-captain with another member. She called me immediately and was very excited. I remember her saying, "It's up to you, but you are a leader, and I think you will do better leading your own team." This was huge to me because she was saying she believed in me. I had zero experience in the contest, but she saw something in me that inspired her confidence in me, and that inspired me.

The Challenge set me on the path of leadership within the KBC community. I like to learn by doing, and it was a ton of work. As most captains do, I became very invested timewise, emotionally, and mentally. My team became my baby for two months, and I am a competitor, so I wanted to show up strong for them.

We had a great team. I liked that the team was a mix of people outside of KBC and a good balance of men and women. Andrew (Kelly's husband) was actually on that team. I don't know if Kelly put him on that team on purpose. It was neat because it was my first time meeting Andrew, and it gave me a chance to see him also step up in a role you don't usually see him in around KBC. I was a new captain, and we had many new people on our team. Andrew had done the contest before; he might've been the only one on our team who was not a rookie.

Andrew stepped up and said, "OK, we've got to do these things to compete." It was interesting because I could tell my husband all day long to eat this, eat that, and he wouldn't listen to me. But when Andrew spoke up, he loved it, and we had a lot of guys on the team, so it was great to have Andrew speak more directly to them. The challenge was a real growing experience for me, and after being a stay-at-home mom for over a decade, it gave me something to focus on outside of my family.

Kelly called me out of the blue a few months after the contest. I was still taking classes regularly and would often stay after with a few friends and help Kelly pack up the equipment in the van. The lot was my happy place, and I loved the energy Kelly poured into every class and everyone who showed up. I remember thinking, *Why is she calling me? Have I done something wrong?* I remember her saying, "I have this idea, and I want to talk to you about it."

She explained that many "nutrition" companies with food plans and supplements consisting of highly processed foods were starting to market to many of our bootcampers. Kelly knew that wasn't a good thing, but she didn't have an alternative to offer people regarding nutrition coaching. She said, "I've seen everything you're doing with nutrition, taking care of your son and your whole family. Would you be interested in getting professional nutrition credentials and helping with nutrition coaching for KBC?"

It was an immediate *yes* from me! I think I started the coursework the next day and worked relentlessly over the summer to complete it.

At this point, before "manifesting," this was a mainstream concept, but I remember lying in bed at night thinking I wanted to be an instructor with KBC. I could do that. Of course, I never told anyone this dream, but it was starting to come alive.

A couple of months later, I remember sitting in Kelly's home with a few other members she wanted to become coaches, and she shared that she wanted to expand the offerings beyond outdoor classes and start Camp U as a higher touch, more comprehensive small group training coaching program. Jodi, Erica, Jen, and I would all be learning and coaching fitness, and then I would do all the nutrition assessments. In

August 2015, I did my first nutrition consultation with Julie White, one of the first Camp U participants. Julie is a breast cancer survivor, had gone through a double mastectomy, and was getting back to workouts and wanted help with her nutrition. She was my case study for my certification.

Even though I had a good understanding of nutrition science, coaching was challenging for me. I had to learn many aspects of behavior change on the job. I remember being very freaked out at how often people would cry or get emotional in meetings. I thought I was there just to talk about food. It took me a while to realize how interconnected food is to every part of our well-being. I had textbook knowledge, but I had to learn on the job how to apply that knowledge to the real world and real people. And sometimes, I was making it up as I went along. It was tough, but I just kept doing the work and putting in the practice and found I loved helping people.

I was also coaching Camp U at the same time. I would show up and help Kelly out, but I was beyond intimidated. She has a powerful presence, and even though I was an accomplished student, I did not know the first thing about coaching fitness. To me, Kelly was such a master instructor that I felt like a big imposter next to her, and I remember thinking, *Maybe I'm not cut out for this.* It felt like learning to preach in front of the pope.

I put a lot of pressure on myself to be perfect from the get-go and did not give myself the grace to not be great at something. I got yelled at by Kelly a few times; I cried, I would take hours to plan a single workout, and then I would stress over whether it was good enough. But I was making progress.

Between Kelly and Jodi, who had been working with Kelly for a few years, I started to learn how to receive constructive feedback. "This was great, but hey, why don't you try this?" And that helped build my confidence. Once I stopped overthinking it all, I relaxed enough to start enjoying the coaching and got to the point where I thought I could do it on my own. In the summer of 2016, I earned my group fitness certification. I still remember my very first class; it was one of Kelly's classes out at the lot, and she needed a last-minute sub. I don't think I've ever been so nervous, but it went well, and I had a new love.

That September, I got my first regular class on the KBC schedule. It was Thursday at 4:30 pm, and we called it the teacher's class because that was mainly who came at that time of day. Kelly said, "I want you to come up with a word for what you want that class to represent." My word was fun. I grew up in a family of teachers and was a teacher before having children, and I knew that by Thursday at 4:30 p.m., teachers just wanted to let go and have some fun. Kelly said that was perfect and not to stress about the exercises. "Just make it fun!" And honestly, I can say that class is still fun nine years later.

That began my journey as a nutrition coach and fitness instructor at KBC. Since then, both the company and my role have expanded exponentially. This growth has been very organic, and I credit Kelly for allowing her team to find their own path and pursue what speaks to them. I have created classes that focus on choreography and my love for music. As a coach, I have discovered a passion for helping women become the strongest and healthiest versions of themselves.

Kelly emphasizes prioritizing the process over the outcome or final goal. This approach reflects our understanding of success, which values consistent effort and being present. Kelly says to Just Show Up, which resonates with me as a student and coach. A few years back, Kelly gifted me a jacket with the slogan "Show up, work hard, and get better," and it still hold special meaning for me.

The most significant benefit of being a part of this community as both a member and instructor is the sense of belonging it provides. As you grow older, finding a sense of belonging becomes increasingly difficult. I still have fond memories of the community that was created at the fitness center where I worked in high school and of the teams I was on in high school and college. It is rewarding and comforting to have somewhere you can Just Show Up as yourself and instantly be a part of something.

Kelly's Take

The first thing I want to acknowledge about Amy's story is that despite her initial doubt, she took it as a sign when multiple people suggested she try out a class even though she didn't think it was what she was looking for. I do not believe any part of her story is a coincidence; she was meant to serve our community significantly, and we were meant to work together. Amy came up with the name Inergy for the studio. We were on a "walk and talk" brainstorming names, and I said I wanted to bring the energy of the outside in. She responded, "Inergy."

Next is how much I trust and respect her. Starting with my desire for my husband to be on her contest team. I knew she was intelligent, strategic, and a clear communicator with great energy. She was also competitive in all the right ways. Andrew is discerning but helpful, and I knew she would be a leader he would respect. I believed they could learn from each other, and the team would benefit from her energy and creativity and his insight into the Winter Challenge.

I've been in the fitness industry for three decades, and the marketing of diets and "weight loss programs" that I believe move your health in the wrong direction have been vast. I wanted to protect our members from wasting their time and money. I'm very sensitive to how vulnerable people are when it comes to their weight and body composition. They're desperate for change, and the conflicting messages of the dieting industry have always disturbed me. I knew Amy would stay true to her core beliefs and values that aligned with mine. I knew she was the solution to a problem that many of our members were facing.

I wonder if many people know why I started Camp U. It all began when one of my friends expressed concern about his wife and wanted her to start exercising. However, he didn't think my large classes would suit her style. During that conversation, I came up with the idea of a small group training program that would be highly personalized. I knew that this new offering would require me to expand my team. It was also a test product for a higher-priced service. While I could easily attract hundreds of people to join my affordable outdoor classes, the question was whether people would be willing to pay more for a premium program. I realized that to open an indoor space, I would have to charge almost double what I was currently charging. I created Camp U to cater to the needs of a specific person. As I learned from my bootcamp experience, if one person has a need, likely others do too.

I also appreciate Amy's honesty in sharing the "Camp U training program." I needed to learn how to share my leadership role. My teammates assisted me with the Saturday bootcamp, but allowing someone else to coach and be the group leader was also a process for me. I had great trust in the people leading Camp U and their skills, but when it came to programming, I knew what I wanted it to look and feel like, and my expectations were very high.

I don't remember yelling, but if I did, it was because I knew she had what it takes. I'm super passionate about my baby, KBC, and inviting others to take ownership was a vast and challenging step. I'm grateful for Amy's grace. Camp U was also a new program for me. I knew how

I wanted it to feel, but I needed to figure out how to get it there. I can be rough when I am unsure of myself. My defense mechanism is to make it the most critical thing and treat it like gold. I am not always my best self in these situations, but I think I have grown here, too, as I have gained confidence and experience.

Amy also gives a great example of the concept of a dream team. I failed to give her the confidence she needed, even though I thought the world of her as a student and in becoming a coach. Jodi stepped up to bridge that gap. The dream team idea is that we complement each other instead of competing. The group fitness and coaching space can be competitive and cutthroat, but we are all unique, and I genuinely believe that we value and appreciate each other's gifts and are all on the same team to help our members look and feel great.

Something about Amy's story stands out; she kept trying to learn. Knowledge truly is power when it comes to getting better at your craft, and I always (even when she was a student) found her to be very coachable, eager to learn, and confident to express that she has her way of processing things.

As I added new members to my team, I realized that to expand, I needed to empower them to take ownership of their program. This meant some things would turn out differently from what I had envisioned. I soon realized that my strength was not in coaching others to become great trainers but in identifying star students who were confident and skilled enough to develop their vision and style. I'm grateful to Amy, Jen, and Erica for allowing me to learn on the job, just as they were doing. I realized this because I believe in treating others the way I want to be treated. I had always enjoyed creating my processes but had to allow my new team members to do the same.

Amy embodies KBC's ethos of gradual, organic growth and making a positive impact. She introduced three signature workouts to Inergy and successfully attracted a large number of attendees both in person and via Zoom. She also created group nutrition programs that are results-oriented, educational, realistic, and fun.

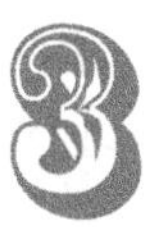

Stay in Your Lane

Where we come from matters. The people surrounding us in our early years help form who we will become. Losing my father in 2008 was a pivotal moment. His influence, even after his passing, guides my choices every day. My dad, Larry Spraragen, epitomized strength and resilience. He was the rock of our family, exuding a sense of power and control. Though he seemed unapproachable sometimes, his wisdom and street smarts were undeniable. Despite his tough exterior, his generosity and commitment to family and community were unwavering. Beneath his tough exterior, a softer side valued honesty, fairness, and protecting his family.

Looking back now, it's easy for me to see my dad as my hero and to admire his toughness and commanding presence. But growing up, I viewed him with fear and confusion, unable to comprehend his strict and demanding nature. He wasn't one to dole out compliments or tell you he was proud, yet I constantly sought his approval.

While my father never used words of affirmation, he repeatedly said a few things to me over the years that I now consider very valuable. One of his recurring remarks was about me being such a Pollyanna. I didn't understand what it meant when he said this to me. In context, he was calling me idealistic, naive, and not in touch with reality. I later learned that characteristics typically associated with a Pollyanna include having an optimistic outlook, a positive attitude, and the ability to forgive and forget past wrongdoings. Thanks, Dad.

He also said you can't fix other people's problems or situations. I think, in some cases, he was referring to my mom, but I think my mom's illness was a factor in helping me develop healthy boundaries, empathy, and understanding.

During my teenage years, there was a stretch where I perceived my dad as unreasonable, unapproachable, and excessively strict. He had a reputation for being intimidating, and it's fair to say he wasn't very open-minded as a parent. He frequently raised his voice at us, meted out harsh punishments, and boasted about his ability to catch us misbehaving because he had done it all before. His approach instilled fear in us, yet we still found ways to get into trouble and make mistakes.

One vivid memory is how adamant he was about restricting phone use on school nights back in the days before caller ID or internet communication. If the phone rang during dinner, he'd swiftly hang it up without a word, which, looking back, seems amusing now but was distressing at the time, especially if I was hoping a boy would call. My sister, Shanon, seemed the least intimidated by him, and I marveled at how she would try to get away with things. She would route the phone cord into her room at night and talk to her friends. When my dad discovered this, he didn't say a word. He would pull the cord from the wall and retire for the night.

Defying my father always seemed to come with dire consequences for me. I recall one incident in high school when he warned me not to give anyone a ride home due to predicted bad weather. Despite his explicit instruction, I dropped off my cousin on my way back home from an away basketball game on an icy evening. As I entered her driveway, disaster struck when another vehicle skidded into mine on the icy road. This led to an indefinite grounding and the loss of my driving privileges. Once again, my father's advice proved on point, reinforcing his seemingly infallible judgment.

One significant instance where my dad's tough exterior softened occurred when my boyfriend and I drove fourteen hours from North Carolina with a U-Haul to pick up family furniture that they were replacing. My dad had asked if I wanted it for my apartment in North Carolina. As we arrived, my boyfriend, who had never met my father before, stood by my side in the garage, slightly nervous but eager to make a good impression. With his dark sunglasses and year-long dark tan, my dad walked right by him without so much as a glance, leaving an awkward silence in his wake. After giving me a tight embrace, we all entered the house, and my dad eventually acknowledged him. That boyfriend became my husband, and he and my dad formed a strong bond down the road. However, at that moment, my dad would not pretend to like this guy he had never met.

My dad exuded a commanding presence that made some uneasy, yet others found comfort in his aura of control. Kevin, a dedicated Schenectady Hardware & Electric (SHE) employee hired directly from Union Hall as a foreman and promoted to an estimator and project manager to work in the office with my dad, cherished the family-like atmosphere at SHE. He emphasized the team's strength and the camaraderie that distinguished them from other companies.

Kevin shared a memorable anecdote about my dad. Upon seeing a guy leaning against a wall, Larry said, "Fire that guy."

Kevin's response was, "We could, but he doesn't work for us." This became a famous Larry story highlighting his practicality and direct approach, which defined his leadership style.

After I had graduated high school and left home, I trusted his opinion on anything. I always wondered what my dad would think in various situations. When house hunting, relocating to Northern Virginia from Richmond with two small children and one on the way, my husband and I found ourselves torn between two homes, each presenting a distinct set of challenges and opportunities. One was a completed house, offering the comfort of immediate occupancy. At the same time, the other had a larger lot, promising endless possibilities but filled with the complexities of construction and decision-making. When I called my dad, detailing the intricacies of both options, his response was unwavering in its simplicity: "Buy the house with the bigger lot."

To him, the choice was clear. Why settle for anything less than the best? And with that simple yet profound statement, he reaffirmed his unwavering belief in the power of aiming high and seizing the opportunities that lay before us.

This was consistent with my dad's identity and what he taught us. My neighbors became my best friends, the community was perfect for our family, and his intuition was spot on. My dad was street smart. He had unerring intuition when it came to business and life. He did things his way, which typically proved to work in his favor.

He was respected for who he was—described as honest, loyal, demanding, and not averse to risk.

He had a difficult family life. He grew up with divorced parents who had issues of their own.

After high school, he went into the Navy and never talked much about his time overseas in Morocco. He did have what we called "war whoops." He would wake up screaming. Knowing what we know now, it was post-traumatic stress disorder (PTSD).

When he met my mom, he was working as an electrician. He didn't have much. My brother Kendall was born when he was twenty-four, and I was born one year later.

My dad worked his way up as an electrician and saved his money to buy the family business from my grandfather. He grew his small family business into the Capital District's (the metropolitan area surrounding Albany) largest electrical contracting company. He was committed to building up the city of Schenectady, New York. He bought old buildings and brought new life to them. He had a reputation for having the Midas touch, turning derelict property into gold.

He was remembered as a quiet benefactor who generously and without fanfare donated to hospitals, theaters, and community organizations. He was also a demanding boss. When he walked in, people had better be working. He despised laziness and dishonesty. He was rough around the edges, didn't do things to fit in or stand out, and was unapologetically himself.

From the beginning of KBC, I did not overthink things. I would make a decision and move forward with confidence. After the Black Friday Bootcamp, I picked a date to start offering regular Saturday morning workouts, and I started. When it was time to build a team of instructors, I found the right people already in my community and hired them. This is how I operate. I don't always consider it a great business skill or something I learned from my dad. But it is clearly both.

My dad had people who did things for him. He had a go-to person for all of the details of his life. He had strong bonds with his accountant, lawyer, key employees, and trusted friends. While he wasn't quick to let anyone in, he would trust them once he did. He would relinquish control and allow that person to carry out their role.

Dan Sullivan and Benjamin Hardy describe this collaboration skill in their book, "Who, Not How."

"It can be easy to focus on *how*, especially for high achievers who want to control what they can control, which is themselves. It takes vulnerability and trust to expand your efforts and build a winning team. It takes wisdom to recognize that other people are more than capable enough to handle much of the *hows* and that your efforts and contribution (your *hows*) should be focused exclusively where your greatest passion and impact are. Your attention and energy should not be spread thin but purposefully directed where you can experience extreme flow and creativity." My dad mastered staying within his skill set and delegating the rest. I consciously try to emulate this skill in my business and life.

My dad was a man of abundance. He never had a scarcity mindset and believed wholeheartedly in his business and people. At the same time, he was very conservative when it came to expenses in his company. I also have an abundance mindset, but I started with minimal financial investments, growing slowly to meet the needs of my members.

My dad valued people. Once you got to know him, you could see his soft side. I don't let people into my business very freely, but once I do, there is trust and respect. It's important for me to be known as honest and fair, and that came from my dad.

In building KBC, I wanted the right people to feel like they were part of the mission and that this business belongs to them just as much as it does to me. My dad felt the same way about the people in his company.

I also emulate my dad's generosity. I believe that part of the responsibility of being a local business owner is contributing to your community, both financially and with time. I am proud to support schools and philanthropic organizations because my dad always did that.

The most important thing to my father was always his friends and family. My father raised six kids, and we have modeled some of my dad's strong characteristics.

Despite the fact that we were stepbrothers and sisters, I don't typically use the term "step" when referring to my siblings. Kendall and I became a part of this intricate family as a result of our parents' divorce. Each of my family members played a part in making me who I am today.

Shanon and Marc are very close in age to Kendall and me. The four of us attended middle school and high school together. Like typical siblings, we sometimes disagreed, but we also stood up for one another. Chris and Brooke, the two kids my dad and Sheila had together, completed our family.

Sheila, my dad's wife, was undoubtedly his perfect complement. She knew how to calm him down, distract him from situations he didn't handle so well, and, most importantly, make him happy. Sheila has remained the rock of our family and an excellent role model as a mother and a giver for all of us. Our family structure was unique and challenging, but Dad and Sheila made it work beautifully.

I learned so much from my dad. One of the most important things he taught me is **Just to Be Yourself**. I don't try to be something I'm not; I focus on what I do best and what lines up with my passion. This translates into a simple concept of **Stay in Your Lane**.

Follow your own passion. Don't worry about what other people are doing or what they'll think of what you're doing. Just do your own thing.

If it doesn't light you up, don't do it. Consider why you like it when you see somebody else doing something that speaks to you. Ask yourself what part of that could be incorporated to enhance what you're doing. Learn from others, but ultimately find what lights you up. Then do that thing.

If it's not your thing to do, there's always someone else who can do it. When I add a new team member at KBC, it's usually because that person has something unique to offer. Having a diverse team of instructors allows us to stay in our own lanes. They can serve who they're best equipped to serve, and I can continue to do what lights me up.

Stay in Your Lane

Follow your own passion. Don't worry about what other people are doing or what they'll think of what you're doing. Just do your own thing. If it doesn't light you up, don't do it.

Just Be Yourself

Don't try to be something you're not. Focus on what you do best and what lines up with your passion.

Heather's Story

I was a dancer growing up. I loved ballet, tap, and jazz. I wasn't interested in traditional exercise like going to the gym or lifting weights. When

I got married, my husband and I started going to the gym together, but I felt lost and unsure what to do. I usually walked on the treadmill and tried lifting weights, but I didn't know what I was doing. After having children, I stopped going to the gym altogether. I remember seeing a bootcamp where groups worked out in a parking lot. It looked pretty intimidating to me. Honestly, I was like, oh my gosh, who would do that?

In 2015, my neighbor started going to KBC, and she invited me to go with her on a bring-a-friend-for-free Saturday. It was intimidating because there were so many people, but everybody was very welcoming. I started attending a couple of classes. I stood in the back of the class; I didn't want people to look at me or laugh because I didn't know what I was doing.

At the end of that same year, I heard Kelly talking about this Winter Challenge; she was looking for people to step up as leaders. In my job, I manage people. I like supporting people and being on a team. So even though I was new to KBC and had never done the challenge, the call for help spoke to me. I'll always remember contacting Kelly; I didn't know her well then. I shared that I might be interested in being a challenge leader. And so she's like, "All right, well, let's get on the phone." I'm like, oh, gosh, what have I gotten myself into?

So we got on the phone, and she asked me why I wanted to take on the challenge and why I wanted to be a leader. My why was that I wanted to meet people and that I liked being on a team and helping others. It was a very short call. And she was like, "OK, you're a captain."

All the leaders met at her house to learn about the logistics of that year's challenge. I felt very supported by the other captains, who had all done the challenge before, and Kelly expressed that she believed in me.

During the challenge, all the teams held events. Our team, Watch Me, organized a workout event that I led. I created a choreographed dance routine to our theme song for the warm-up session. A heavy snowfall occurred the week before the event and people were cooped up in their homes. Luckily, on the day of our event, the sun was shining, and everyone was excited to be outside and together. I stood before my team, looking out at the massive crowd of bootcampers. Everyone seemed to be enjoying themselves, and the energy was upbeat and fun. It was a far cry from when I used to stand at the back, not wanting to be seen.

My teammates and I formed a great bond while working together. I'm still close with my former teammates and enjoy meeting them at the lot or Inergy. My husband, an artist, helped me design the logos for our team. Although he prefers going to the gym, he also tinkered with the bootcamp and is very supportive of the KBC community.

Kelly is an encouraging leader who always shows gratitude toward those who step up. During Winter Challenge parties, she makes it a point to acknowledge and thank each captain. Her gestures are so heartwarming that they motivate people to do it again. One year, Kelly asked all the teammates to write a letter to their captain, thanking or acknowledging them. I still have those letters. They meant so much to me and were such beautiful gestures.

My father passed away almost five years ago. Kelly had the opportunity to meet him at that challenge event. Whenever we spoke, my father always asked me if I had gone to bootcamp that morning. He was fascinated by it. My mother also attended the event because I talked about it so much. Both of them were amazed that I would work out in thirty-degree weather. My father, an entrepreneur at heart, was fascinated by Kelly's story, and I know he would have loved to read her book. He took pictures at the event, and my mother still can't get over the experience.

When my father passed away, Kelly reached out to me. She knew I was out of town and that I would deliver the eulogy. I will never forget when she sent me a text message that said, "Make sure that you look your best today for your dad." I did not feel like putting on any make-up, doing my hair, or dressing up. However, I couldn't stop thinking about Kelly's message that morning. So I dressed, put on some makeup, and did my hair nicely. I wanted to make my dad proud. I delivered his eulogy without crying, and at the end, I realized that I spoke clearly without the typical filler words that I would use when I was nervous.

Kelly's Take

Heather's story has so many significant layers. It's important that people feel welcome and that there's an opportunity for them to be in the KBC community to grow beyond just fitness gains and body composition changes. I understand how intimidating it can be to start, but when somebody is confident to join and stick with the outdoor program over the colder months, they are typically capable of much more.

When Heather asked me about being a Winter Challenge leader, I didn't even need to have that phone call; she had already shown me her character and determination by showing up for class. She is a great student, a leader, and a team player. If you have something in your heart, you will find a way to make it happen. Her why was the perfect answer.

I love the irony of going from not being a gym person and hiding in the back to standing up in front of one hundred people to doing a warm-up for a workout and naming her team Watch Me. One piece of advice I give my clients when they are trying to accomplish something is to attach it to something they already like. When Heather came to bootcamp, she might have been surprised that we moved to the music (just like in dance), and I think it was brilliant that she took many of us out of our comfort zone with a dance-inspired warm-up after she had stepped out of her comfort zone to come to bootcamp and lead a Challenge team.

I started bootcamp to honor my father, so anytime a parent of a bootcamper takes an interest, it is an honor. Heather had talked so much about her dad, maybe because I had shared so much about my father. I was touched when he came to the event with Heather's mom to take pictures and show support. Heather had significantly impacted the community, and I got an opportunity to share how adored and appreciated she was with her parents.

One of the many topics discussed in the KBC Community is legacy. Every year at the Black Friday Bootcamp, an annual event since 2008, I used to share a bit about my dad. However, at some point, I decided that I would like the members of the KBC Community to share something they learned from *their* parents or a memorable experience they had with a parent who passed away. At the end of the Black Friday Bootcamp, each participant who wanted to speak shared a lesson they learned or something they admired about their parents. Some people are not ready to share because the pain of losing a parent is too raw. Sadly, over the years, this has become a mutual bond for many of us, and it's also a great reminder for those with a living parent to be grateful.

I'm grateful that Heather remembered our text exchange on the day of her father's funeral. When I met Dan, her father, it was clear that Heather was the apple of his eye. Even though it might have seemed odd, I thought to myself on the day of my own father's funeral that I wanted to look my best for the important people in my dad's life who would be there. Despite my devastation, I wanted to make my dad proud. Focusing on that got me through the day and was my way of helping Heather.

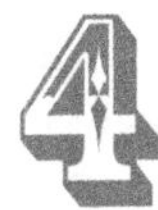

You Are a Dreamer

Growing up with a mother who battled bipolar disorder, my childhood was a roller coaster of emotions and uncertainty. Each hospitalization left me wondering when she would return and in what state. It was a challenging time, but looking back, I realize it laid the foundation for my life's mission. It took me a long time to acknowledge it, but I believe my calling to coach people toward physical and mental strength stems from those early experiences.

Despite her struggles, my mother was a beacon of creativity and talent. She was passionate about many things and would go all in on whatever she did. Everything was a project. If she was going to cook, a full day's event. Sewing, she would pull all-nighters.

Music was her happy place. Unfortunately, when she became engrossed in writing songs or playing guitar, it usually meant she was getting sick.

Her music was unique, and she became prolific at writing when she was sick. The songs had meaning and were sometimes her own stories. One of her songs refers to a trip she was on (she was hospitalized), and she sings, "I got to see my babies. This trip's driving me crazy." We were her babies, and I always liked knowing that part was about me.

There was a time when she hosted a weekly country music jam session at her home. Everyone was welcome to join in regardless of their musical talent and experience. She often had as many as twenty people playing along and even more there just to listen. I know she inspired and encouraged many people to love music and left a legacy.

My mother's journey taught me the importance of authenticity and following your passion, even in the face of adversity. Her unwavering commitment to her dreams left a lasting impression on me despite the challenges she faced.

Inheriting her passion and creativity, I've channeled these traits into my own endeavors, particularly in my business. Designing themed workouts and events allows me to tap into my vision and bring it to life with energy and excitement.

Through it all, I've learned that resilience isn't about avoiding challenges but embracing them as growth opportunities. My mother's illness may have been a part of our story, but it taught me valuable lessons about perseverance, compassion, and the power of pursuing your dreams.

My lifelong mission has been to empower people to believe in themselves and focus on what they can control. I want individuals to understand their direct influence on their well-being. To me, the strength that you get from a workout transfers to every aspect of your life. Being in check with your eating and proud of the foods that you choose to consume is a life hack that can serve you through any stage and season. My early experiences with my mom helped shape my mission. It led me to be authentically myself. A hard worker. A person who gets things done. A person who strives to serve others and bring others together in the community.

My mom was funny. She would make up silly songs and rhymes and laugh really hard at her own jokes. She was sometimes almost childlike when she talked to the squirrels and the birds. My friends liked being around her; in high school, she would cook delicious food and make us laugh. My friends were also there for me when my mom got sick. They would help me manage the damage, love, and talk me through the hard times. These friends are still an essential part of my life today, and that is probably why I value and prioritize the people in my life and try to be there for others. Somebody was always there for me. I never felt alone.

What made my mom unique was that she always did what she wanted. She followed her passion instead of rules and expectations. The best way to describe her is **authentic.** She possessed strong values. She always upheld integrity, respected authority, and was honest and pragmatic when her mental health was stable. This made the extreme aspects of her personality, during episodes, particularly alarming. I guess that's why they call it bipolar disorder.

She was respected for her talents and gifts, teaching others to cook, sew, and play guitar. She had friends and admirers. While her sickness strained some relationships, supporters were always in her corner, offering help and compassion.

Despite frequent hospitalizations, she never gave up and let failure or roadblocks take away from her dreams. One of the lines in her best song, "Silver Dollar Woman," was, "**You Are a Dreamer** girl, yeah, you know you got that right."

No matter the devastation, the debt, or the difficulties, my mom always came back. Sometimes, it took a long time. She would get overwhelmed and depressed, but eventually, she was back to living and dreaming.

Some of the stories of cars, furniture, auction hauls, and real estate that she purchased during her mania are unbelievable. But she did it. It was a mess to clean up and often cost a lot of time and money. My favorite (not really) was when she took a full-page ad in the Schenectady Gazette running for mayor. Her delusions were very real. When she was in a manic state, all of her passion and energy came through, but she also became mean and difficult to deal with, which was very different from the person she was.

Growing up with a parent facing mental illness, I learned firsthand the importance of resilience and self-belief. Witnessing the struggles my mother faced, I realized the significance of mental strength in overcoming adversity. Instead of allowing her challenges to define me, I chose to see them as opportunities for growth and self-discovery.

My journey taught me that resilience is not about being immune to difficulties but how we respond to them. We can navigate even the toughest situations by embracing challenges with a positive mindset and unwavering faith in our abilities.

Through my own experiences, I discovered the power of empathy and emotional expression as tools for coping and healing. By allowing myself to feel and process my emotions, I found the strength to move forward and overcome obstacles.

My story serves as a reminder that resilience is not a trait we're born with but a skill that can be developed and nurtured over time. By sharing our experiences and supporting one another, we can empower others to cultivate resilience and thrive in adversity.

My relationship with my mom, as all relationships do, evolved over time. In the years before my mom died, ALS had taken over her body. At one point, we were told she wouldn't make it through the summer. She lived through three more summers. Two years before her death, hospice was brought in to make her last few months comfortable. She lived on for years instead of months. Despite recommendations of tube feeding shortly after diagnosis, my brother and I fed her fried chicken and Chinese food until the last four months of her life. She had an incredibly strong will to live. She wanted more time with the people she loved.

While spending time with her during this illness, I was given an opportunity to see my mother in a different light. After a lifetime of being angry at her for who she was, I gained a new genuine respect and admiration for her resilience and strength. She never complained about the disease that was robbing her of everything that she loved to do. She focused on being grateful for the people around her and her goal of hearing her songs played on the radio. She asked me to help her fulfill her dream of having her music played on the radio. Despite countless emails, phone calls, and letters, I failed at this mission. In her determination, she held onto her dream, and miraculously, a DJ who became a fan of her music through one of her musician friends helped turn that aspiration into reality.

Excerpts from her favorite song, "Silver Dollar Woman," echoed the sentiments of her unwavering spirit:

"All I wanted to do was to hear the country music play."

"Suddenly, the magic filled the air."

"You're a dreamer woman for sure, yeah, you got that right."

In her perseverance and unwavering optimism, my mother's legacy lives on, a testament to the power of resilience and the pursuit of dreams against all odds.

Be Authentic

To be true to your own personality, values, and spirit, regardless of the pressure that you're under to act otherwise. To be honest with yourself and others.

Meg's Story

I met Kelly twenty years ago when we first moved into our neighborhood. We became friends, and she encouraged me to join Olympus, one of the gyms where she taught. I had never really exercised before. I danced growing up, and then I would do Jazzercise for a little bit with friends, but I was never consistent. I wasn't a regular exerciser and did not consider myself an athlete.

I started doing her classes at Olympus. I would show up in my big baggy outfits, and my face would be bright red by the end of the class, but somehow, she got me hooked. When her father passed away, she shared that her family was doing a half marathon race in Las Vegas on her dad's birthday. She asked if I wanted to come, and I said I could never run a half marathon. I can't even run a mile.

I said, "I'll go and cheer you guys on."

And she said, "No, you're not allowed to go if you don't do the race. Meg, I think you could do this. Hop on a treadmill. If you can run for a mile, you can totally do a half marathon."

So I hopped on the treadmill, set it to a nice easy pace, and was shocked that I could do a mile. I mean, I was shocked. So I said, "OK, all right, well, maybe I'll do this." And so I started training, and I did it. I ran the entire half marathon and couldn't believe it. I crossed the finish line and sobbed. One of the things about Kelly that makes her successful is that she believes in people before they believe in themselves. She makes them think, oh, maybe I can do this. I've been with her since starting KBC and always helped her behind the scenes. I loved what she was doing. I adored the community that she was creating. I appreciated the changes that I was seeing and the impact she was making on so many lives.

I was grateful for the community and wanted to show support, so I cheered her on behind the scenes, helping make name tags or filing. We used to have sheets of paper used at bootcamp when she would have different challenges. People would find their folders with their sheets of paper and write down the scores.

It's unbelievable to think that I stuck with the workouts. I had never been consistent with exercise because I didn't enjoy it. I'm social and like connecting and spending time with Kelly, so that was the initial hook. She would say, are you coming to class? And I'd say OK. Being friends with Kelly created accountability.

And then I noticed that my face wasn't getting as red. The classes started getting a little easier. When you go regularly, you build these relationships with the other people who attend the classes. So you start having this sense of community. Even while teaching at Olympus, Kelly has always created this sense of community, cheering for each other and celebrating birthdays in class. Whatever it is, she makes people feel special.

I was there for the first Black Friday Bootcamp, and my husband and I were regulars at Saturday bootcamp. When she started adding weekday classes, I came to those too!

In 2017, after Inergy opened, I began the fitness professional certification process. Kelly had always taught all the classes herself. I saw a need for her to expand her team, and I wanted to help people the way she's helped me.

Before I was certified, I was starting with the Retro Program (the two-day-a-week fifty-five-plus workout that Jodi, one of Kelly's original team members, initiated). I helped Jodi as her assistant.

When I finished my certification, I took over one of the days.

As needs opened up, I added a few morning classes to my schedule, and in 2023, I became certified in yoga. Now, I teach seven classes a week and try to help with subbing.

Kelly says that if you want it badly enough, you'll find a way to make it happen. I've gained confidence through KBC; it started with not thinking I could run a half marathon and then crossing the finish line and seeing people's transformations in the bootcamp community. It makes you feel like anything is possible if you just find something that works for you and stick with it. Even the slightest acknowledgment or encouragement makes a difference in people's day, life, and confidence. You just never know how what you say impacts someone.

So many students have become consistent with exercise at KBC because people know that Kelly cares about them coming to workouts and about their success. I have encouraged Kelly to write a book because her story can resonate with anyone. She started small, in a parking lot, and her passion was helping people. Kelly would say I just want to have enough people there to cover the cost of the babysitter. So if that were five people, she was thrilled with it. She wanted to make a difference for those five people but didn't want it to impact her family negatively.

So for people trying to create this dream themselves, the key is starting small, being passionate, genuinely caring, gradually growing, listening to your customers as to what they need, and then slowly building on your own success.

Kelly's Take

Meg's story highlights a massive part of my reason for writing a book. One of the messages that I want to share (especially those who are taking care of the needs of others and not their own) is that the time you invest in your health will return to you and those you care about and serve. Meg is the most generous person I have ever met and constantly gives to others in countless ways, the biggest being her time. She extends herself to her community, family, and friends and thinks nothing of being on boards, PTAs, president of service organizations, and bringing meals to strangers. However, when we met, she wasn't taking care of herself.

She was the queen of looking for a quick fix to lose weight, but I don't think she understood what being healthy looked like. From Meg, I learned to think more about service and the needs of others, and from me, she discovered that you will be far better equipped to take care of others if you prioritize your health and fitness.

The real gem of this story is Meg's desire to give back to KBC and the compound effect of her efforts.

One thing that KBC has created organically is culture. I believe that part of the strong culture originated from members like Meg, who had a great experience and results and felt the desire to give back. We talk a lot about the Ripple Effect, and having members who understand and support the mission and organically become a leader is the foundation of this.

The idea of becoming an instructor for KBC was her own. I knew she would be a great coach because I know how much work she puts into everything she does, and one of the critical criteria I have for my team is genuinely caring about the success of our members. The addition of regular yoga classes has been a gift to the community, and the one class I prioritize in my fitness regime is her yin yoga class.

Her story of slow organic growth parallels that of KBC itself, emphasizing the importance of starting small, being passionate, creating programs to meet the expanding needs of our members, and genuinely caring about others' success.

Everything Matters

Following my parents' divorce, my brother and I began to settle into our new surroundings. In addition to a new family, house, and school, I also acquired a newspaper route. I wasn't actually old enough to have my own paper route. My older sister, Shanon, and I became partners. Having a paper route is a big deal. We had to deliver paper seven days a week. People were very picky about exactly where they wanted their paper. Winters are brutal in NY, and the paper had to be delivered by 6:30 a.m.

As if that wasn't enough, we also had to collect payment. We had to knock on doors and ask people to pay us. Then, we had to pay the route manager every two weeks—regardless of whether we could catch people at home who were willing to answer the door and pay us in cash. This was long before autopay started, and there were no options to pay by credit card. Sometimes we had to use our own funds to pay the route manager, Mr. Dingly.

Collecting was my first experience with customer service. Some clients invited us in and offered us a beverage. Others would clearly be home and avoid opening the door. In some situations, we received very generous tips. Some customers would pay ahead, but others waited impatiently as I fumbled through our money pouch to return the seventy-five cents in change.

My favorite house belonged to an older couple. There was a very long driveway and a table underneath a big tree in the backyard. They used to leave a brown bag on the table filled with butterscotch candies and a handwritten note. That house was nicknamed the butterscotch lady. Other nicknames included nice people house, house that smells, green door house, name of doghouse, and others.

Speaking of dogs: Wheezy! Wheezy was a little dog that lived on the end of our route. He would chase us. If we were on our bikes, we were fine. But being on foot near Wheezy's house was scary. We never collected payment at Wheezy's house, so I guess they got the paper for free.

We had a big route. It was actually two routes combined. Sometimes Shanon and I would collaborate on holding the bag, folding the paper, and using our cheat sheet to determine if they wanted the paper in the mailbox, between the doors, or under the mat. Other mornings, we would divide and go in different directions, meeting in the middle.

This whole process seems pretty primitive today. But the real glitch was that customers had a punch card that indicated how much they owed. They kept the card at their home. Nothing stopped them from using their hole punch and declaring that they already paid. We had a book to keep track of it all, but I'm unsure if we ever really did that part of the paper route business.

And now, the best part of having a paper route. A few mornings, when it was raining really hard or the snow made walking unbearable, I would wake my dad and ask him to drive us. He usually said no. But a few times, he caved, and we would drive from house to house in a heated car, just popping out to place the paper in the right spot. Those mornings were glorious.

Remember that Shanon was my ticket to managing a route. After a while, she didn't like getting up early on cold mornings. Eventually, she decided to retire. I needed a new partner. Next up was my stepbrother, Marc. I loved collecting with Marc because he had a story about every house and its people. Marc and I happily shared the route for several years. We made a good team.

At some point, Marc too decided it was too much hassle and not enough reward. My third business partner was my neighbor and friend, Kris. By this point, I was old enough to have the route in my name, and customers started to appreciate my loyalty and service. Christmas was a jackpot! People would come to the door with the money for the paper and a holiday card. We saved all the cards until we got home and would open them one by one, stacking up the piles of dollar bills.

As I got older, I moved on to other jobs and activities. But my early experience managing my paper route planted the seed of a lesson I still adhere to today. **Everything matters**. The work I did on those cold mornings mattered. It mattered to my partners. It mattered to my customers. It mattered to me.

You'll soon read about other jobs I had in my early years, long before I became a business owner. But delivering papers with my sibling was my first job: the first time I was paid for a task, the first time I had customers who depended on me. My belief that everything you do matters started to develop during this work and would strengthen with each job and responsibility I have taken on.

Delivering the newspaper on foot at the crack of dawn in upstate NY, waiting tables, babysitting, showing up to sports practice, being a good friend, trying hard in school—those were all very important things, and I took them very seriously. My friends would say, "It's just

Friendly's," or "This test doesn't even count." But there's something about doing your best all the time. It matters.

In "Girl, Wash Your Face," Rachel Hollis says, "Friends, it's not about the goal or the dream you have. It's about who you become on your way to that goal." Every action you take reflects who you are, but more importantly, who you are becoming. All the little things you do along the way and all the giant things you do matter.

I have always liked to work. I like feeling productive, especially if it involves feeling significant or adding value. I think one of the reasons that I'm a good business owner is that I have always treated every job I have had like it was my business. Every job mattered. Every day of work, every task—it all mattered. And the same is true for you: every decision you make, every action you take is leading toward something. It all matters.

Everything Matters

Everything you do matters. Even the smallest, seemingly unimportant tasks should be done to the best of your ability.

The process matters just as much as what you've accomplished.

Margery's Story

I've been attending Kelly's classes since her very first class. I was a mother of three little girls; my youngest was only three. I was looking for a workout place other than waking up early to run with my neighbors. I played soccer all my life and loved being outside. Kelly's classes seemed like a perfect fit. Kelly asked us to bring our weights and a mat and promised we would get what we came for.

It's been fifteen years since I started attending Kelly's classes, and I've gained much more than I expected. Even though many things have changed over the years, Kelly still consistently asks for feedback from the community. Despite our diverse backgrounds, we all enjoy being part of something bigger than ourselves. I still eagerly look forward to attending the classes and seeing familiar faces.

One thing she has taught the bootcamp community is vulnerability, turning your struggle into your strength. If we lean on each other, we will ultimately be stronger.

People in the community have immense faith and trust in Kelly, and when you see positive changes happening and feel welcomed somewhere, it makes you want to return. This is what Kelly does for people in the KBC community and beyond.

Kelly always finds a way to uplift and bring people out of their darkness. I lost my older sister about a year and a half ago. Losing her left me feeling shattered and alone. Unfortunately, I'm not the only one in our community who has experienced such a loss. However, I have noticed that Kelly possesses a unique ability to uplift people during these difficult times. Everyone in the community knows of my love for my sister and how hard it was for me to cope with her loss. Unsurprisingly, this special community rallied around me, giving me the love and support to persevere. Kelly has built something incredibly special. It's not just the best workout in town. You are surrounding yourself with the best people in town.

Kelly's Take

You are best equipped to serve the person that you once were. The creation of the KBC community brought me out of the dark. Building a strong workout community from the ground up was my way of honoring my father and channeling my sadness. When KBC helps others during the most challenging times, I'm reminded of how powerful I always thought my father was and how he lives on through me and my community.

As you read Margery's story, you may have noticed that she tends to divert the focus away from herself. She is the kind of person who consistently goes out of her way to assist and support others, even if it means making personal sacrifices. Margery's contributions to welcoming new members and making them feel comfortable are essential to KBC's culture. Founding members like Margery set standards that have become a significant part of why many feel like they are part of a community.

Margery was very athletic, fit, and strong when she began working out fifteen years ago. One could argue that she is now physically stronger and has better stamina, but most impressive is that she has aged in reverse. She is a shining example of the benefits of consistent effort and dedication to fitness. She exemplifies the belief that you get out what you put in and that a workout is never just a workout.

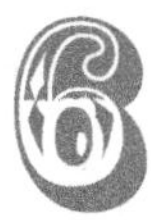

Start Something,
Then Find Your Passion

Have you ever heard of Friendly's?

You know, the place to get Reese's Pieces sundaes, the ones with hot fudge, marshmallow, and peanut butter sauce topped with whipped cream, chocolate sprinkles, Reese's Pieces, and a cherry on top.

Friendly's is a wonderful place that brings happiness to families, older adults who live alone, middle schoolers after the big dance, and hungry early morning workers. This bustling environment is where my adaptability and communication skills started to develop. I began to understand the dynamics of both business operations and customer satisfaction. It might seem odd that a fitness professional who spends her days helping others make sound choices about their health and wellness would include Friendly's in her book. But stay with me.

I filled out an application to be a waitress at Friendly's on April 5, 1988. I sat at the counter and included my four-plus years of experience with my paper route and my babysitting resume. When I handed the application back to the manager, he asked me to sit down. He looked down at my application, and he looked back up at me and said, "You're only fifteen."

You had to be sixteen to work at Friendly's.

I replied, "I'll be sixteen tomorrow."

Friendly's became my happy place. I loved being a waitress. It was a small restaurant with only three servers working during the busiest shifts. It was a challenging and demanding job, but that was OK with me. Some people came in to get ice cream, but we also offered breakfast, lunch, and dinner. Breakfast was my favorite shift to work. On Sunday mornings, I would open up the restaurant at 6:00 a.m. For the first hour, it was usually just the cook and me, so I would run the entire front of the house, seating, taking orders, specking out the food, delivering food, making drinks, cashing customers, clearing the tables, and getting them ready for the next guests.

It was at Friendly's that I learned how to serve customers. I learned to bring crayons and crackers to young children, remember special requests for my regular customers, and go out of my way to create a fun and memorable experience.

I also learned that I needed to be extra nice to the cooks to get my food out quickly and hot. I would ask them if they needed anything and say, "Wow, that was quick," when the order was ready. It was also important to assist the fountain crew when the line was out the door for ice cream orders.

Friendly's became a place where I got lots of positive recognition and thrived. I was acknowledged for being fast, friendly, and efficient. Customers went out of their way to compliment me, write comment cards, and share positive experiences with the manager. If I messed up an order, I always did whatever I could to make it up to the customer.

My friends would joke that I acted like I owned the place. They weren't wrong. I knew the more efficient the kitchen and the back of the house were, the more tables I could serve in a shift. The more tables I served a shift, the more crumpled one dollar bills I would have in my pouch at night's end.

To say that Friendly's had a significant impact on my life may sound like an exaggeration, but it is true. I worked as a waitress in various restaurants while attending college and graduate school. I gained valuable skills such as empathy, patience, teamwork, and multitasking. I also met some very significant people and learned some invaluable life lessons.

How I went from hiding peanut butter cups under five scoops of ice cream and toppings to becoming a lifer in the health and fitness industry might not make the most sense until you connect the dots.

According to Steve Jobs, "You can't connect the dots until you look back." It's only been in recent years that I've come to understand how my early job experiences were setting me up to own a fitness business. Jobs like the ones I had delivering newspapers and waiting tables offered opportunities to learn, develop, and grow.

Passion is not something that you can brainstorm about. It doesn't live in your head. It lives in your heart. Passion is something you feel when you do it. By taking action, you can start feeling your way to what lights you up.

When I worked at Friendly's, I didn't yet know what my passion would be later in life. I didn't know I would find my passion in helping others fall in love with working toward better health. What I did at Friendly's was start. I just started working and bringing my best to work every day. Along the way, I started to feel my passion for serving others. Sometimes, you have to **Start Something, Then Find Your Passion.**

Later in my life, I had no idea that leading an outdoor workout would energize me. It wasn't until I physically took action for one class that my passion for starting my outdoor fitness business emerged. I wasn't ready to be a waitress; I had no relevant experience, but it was the perfect place to learn and grow.

In the best-selling book, "The 5 Second Rule," Mel Robbins said it best: "Start before you're ready. Don't prepare, begin." When you take action, any action, you can grow and learn along the way. You have the opportunity to discover passion. If you wait until you're ready, you may lose the opportunity to find that passion.

Another key is bringing positive energy to everything you do, even if it is not your favorite thing. Bringing enthusiasm to daily tasks changes your energy and leads to your passion.

When your energy is good, people want to be around you, and good things naturally come your way. When people start an exercise program, I advise finding a way to love it. This might even mean the coffee they get after class, connecting with a friend, or the feeling they have after the workout.

Having a purpose-driven life makes me a happier person. I measure success in what my work has done for the people around me. In all my work experiences, I have always found happiness in creating value for others.

Creating value for others has been my key to personal growth and success, even before I was an entrepreneur looking to build my business. Focusing on what others need pushes you to work harder and with more intention.

At KBC, we have a saying: **Last Set, Best Set**. Our workouts are often organized into sets of exercises that we repeat several times. People show up to workouts for different reasons. However, the one thing they all have in common is that they showed up and started the workout. When the time rolls around for the last set, I hope that it is the best set—a strong finish. It's the best set because they find their passion sometime during the workout. The best set can only happen because you started, because you did the first set. You can finish strong because you started.

Start Something, Then Find Your Passion

Sometimes, you have to take action before you know what your passion is. You just have to start. You might not have a specific plan or even a goal, but you can fall in love with the process.

Last Set, Best Set

In a KBC workout, the final set of exercises should be your best. You should finish strong.

Whatever you do in life, finish strong. To finish strong, you first have to start.

Jenny's Story

Kelly and I are neighbors and friends. In 2008, I took her step class at Gold's Gym where our toddler daughters would play in the child care center together. When Kelly was considering starting her own classes, she had gotten together with a few of us and asked, "Hey, what do you think about if I were to do this outdoor bootcamp on Saturday mornings?" I was one of the ones that suggested doing both the seven o'clock and an eight o'clock because I had little kids and I knew my husband would want to participate as well. Like many other bootcamp couples,

I would take the seven o'clock and come home a few minutes early and my husband would race off to the eight o'clock. Fifteen years later, both of our husbands still take classes together.

After expanding her Saturday bootcamp to include weekday classes, Kelly began contemplating opening an indoor studio. She approached me about teaching barre to complement our existing outdoor training. Given my background in dance and athleticism, coupled with Kelly's praise for my form and posture, I enthusiastically agreed. I obtained my barre instructor certification and started teaching classes in her garage before the indoor studio was ready. That's where my journey as an instructor began. As I started filling in for other classes, I found myself drawn to group fitness in general, not just barre. So I obtained my group fitness instructor credentials and began teaching a variety of classes, finding more passion in cardio and strength training.

Nowadays, I'm teaching several formats, including core fusion and other signature formats that evolved from the needs and wants of our members. It's been a natural evolution. I've never considered myself a fitness enthusiast, and before taking classes with Kelly, I tended to shy away from it. However, I was drawn to KBC's sense of community and camaraderie. What really keeps me engaged now is the community aspect. While I'm still not someone who lives and breathes fitness, I find joy in teaching and witnessing others build confidence and achieve their goals. Without KBC, I'm not sure I'd be as committed to working out regularly. It's the community that keeps me coming back.

I feel that our health, both mine and my husband's, has been significantly affected. Participating in the Winter Challenge each year reminds us of the importance of our eating habits and how they contribute to our well-being beyond just fitness. This yearly routine helps us refocus on nutrition and overall wellness. Just as important, the friendships we've formed through the contest have had an even greater impact on me, and I value the opportunity to reconnect with people who have positively impacted me. Many of these friendships were forged through KBC, and these connections have brought great joy to my life.

Her quotes, like "Get what you came for," have truly resonated with me over time. Even seemingly simple ones, like "you can do anything for a minute," strike a chord with people. It's fascinating how these little sayings continue influencing me and finding their way into my teaching. Her impact and the path she paved seem to reverberate through all the instructors.

Those words also carry through to other aspects of my life, especially when facing a challenging situation. The idea that you can truly accomplish anything, whether for a minute or a mile, resonates with me. I believe her positive energy influences other aspects of my life. On a bad day, just showing up matters. But beyond that, it's not just during workouts with her. There are many instances where I think of Kelly in different situations, and I admire her passion and fierceness. We could all use a bit more of that.

There's something almost magical about how the community comes together, especially when someone new joins. Everyone is so welcoming, and nobody ever feels out of place. It's like this magical bond where the community stands united. I believe Kelly's vision fosters this environment, but she has also inspired others in the community to stand out like her, creating a ripple effect.

Kelly's Take

Listening to Jenny's interview really stirred up my emotions. I wish I could say I had this grand vision of creating a magical community where everyone supported each other and embraced newcomers with open arms. Starting Saturday bootcamp was scary, but when friends like Jenny stepped up and expressed their excitement to participate, along with her husband and other friends wanting to join, I felt a sense of purpose. There was a genuine need, and people appreciated the idea of a once-a-week session that was conveniently located and wouldn't disrupt their family activities for the day. Much of the magic has come from being able to discern the needs of the individuals attending and striving to fulfill those needs.

Jenny is just one of the many individuals who have contributed to the evolution of KBC. Asking her to become an instructor wasn't solely based on her athleticism and dance background. Jenny possesses a natural leadership ability coupled with compassion, and it is evident that she believes that fitness can transform lives, not just for fitness enthusiasts. She was drawn to the sense of community and camaraderie, which is apparent in how she shows up for her students and the team.

The aspect of this story that stands out to me is Jenny's natural progression as a fitness professional. She dedicates considerable effort to meticulously planning her classes, driven by a genuine desire to provide an experience where members feel accomplished and pushed outside their comfort zones. She has grown so much, and I can't help but smile as I read through the plethora of glowing reviews she receives from our members month after month. Her dedication to her craft stems from her joy in witnessing members gain confidence and inner strength through fitness, mirroring the journey I observed her undergo.

Jenny is a perfect example of how "get what you came for" can mean different things at different times. Why she started bootcamp and her why fifteen years later are very different, but what is important is that her why was significant to her.

My husband has always discouraged doing business with friends, but in Jenny's case, she was a friend who became a star student. Identifying students who exemplify the qualities I seek in community leaders may contribute to the robust ripple effect observed within this community.

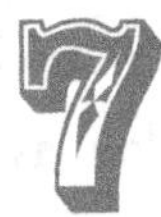

Change the Voice in Your Head

My early experiences with fitness began with organized sports. On the fields, courts, and tracks, I started to learn about the importance of having a coach. I was fortunate to have several coaches who believed in me, encouraged me, and motivated me to succeed. Thirty-five years later, their voices still echo in my mind. Looking back, it's clear that my teenage years were the foundation for me to become a coach and a mentor.

My first experience being on a team was in middle school when I played intramural basketball. Our coach knew that none of us were particularly experienced basketball players, and when we lost badly or never scored a basket, she would say encouraging words that spoke to our efforts and character. She always cheered for us in a loving and nurturing way. Even though I didn't yet have the skills or experience to be the best basketball player, I knew that having a coach and being on a team was my happy place. I loved the practice after school, the bus ride to the game, and the halftime huddle of encouraging words, regardless of the numbers on the scoreboard. We were a group of girls with a common goal of getting better. We lifted each other up. We followed the example of our coach, who wanted us to improve but was happy with who we were at the time.

By high school, I knew I wanted to be an athlete. Most of my close friends planned to play field hockey as we started ninth grade. However, the summer before, I had some exposure to soccer as a guest player, so I decided to try out for the freshman soccer team. Most of the other players had been playing since they were five years old, but I was just getting started. What I lacked in experience, I made up in heart and hustle. I made the team and had a great season my freshman year.

That year, my math teacher was also the head soccer coach. We'll just call him Coach Banana. He was very intimidating. I was petrified of him, and he never seemed interested in me. Now, my best friend Beth, that was another story. Coach Banana loved Beth. He always complimented her, asked about her weekend, and happily declared to the class that Beth was his favorite. After spring break, Coach Banana found out that Beth and I had gone on vacation together. He liked to make jokes during class and asked if Beth stayed in the basement because she was naturally fair, and my skin turned summer brown after one day in the sun. I wouldn't say I liked Coach Banana, but I wanted him to like me. On the first day of school, he told us that if anybody aced the Regents statewide algebra exam, he would call our house. That motivated me. I was so proud when he called my house to congratulate me. That was probably the first and last perfect score I got on a math exam. Even though the school year was over, I assumed that after that, he must like me a little. More importantly, it was a tangible example of the power of setting your mind to a long-term outcome and taking many little actions throughout the year to achieve it. It was a lesson that I would refer to in my mind as an example of the power of putting your mind to something that seems impossible and actually achieving it.

Throughout high school, sports continued to be my happy place. At home, there were lots of things that I couldn't control, and having sports as my focus helped ground me. I loved being on a team and being coached. I also loved knowing that if I worked hard and did what the coaches said, I could improve and make a difference for the team. I also learned that you didn't need to be the best to have an impact or be a leader. Significance was something that I really craved, and the camaraderie of a sports team is where I found it. Belonging and having shared goals within a team made me feel valuable and seen as a person.

I decided to participate in spring track to stay in shape for soccer and basketball. After the first day of practice, the head coach of the varsity team started calling me her five-footer. I had no idea what she was talking about. I was at least five foot seven! Once the season got going, I figured out that she needed a varsity high jumper, and five feet was the height she wanted me to be able to jump over. She believed that I was the girl for the job. Mrs. Cleveland thought I could do something that I didn't even know existed. She gave me a critical mission and the tools to succeed, and she cheered for me during all four years of high school. It was amazing to have someone believe in me and coach me toward success.

Mrs. Cleveland did all sorts of extra things to bring our team together. She made homemade ceramic Smurf figures (a cartoon character in the 90s) to award teammates throughout the season. When we loaded the bus after a travel meet, she would hand every athlete a Twizzler. She recognized everyone instead of always talking about the best people. She talked about PRs (personal records). Maybe not everyone would have a chance to earn first place in an event, but a PR was always possible if you showed up and tried to improve. She also kept a handmade scrapbook of our team pictures, articles, and awards. She delivered these books to any athlete who stayed with track and field all four years.

Even though track and field may be considered an individual sport, Mrs. Cleveland was very strategic about sharing what we needed as far as team points to keep us motivated. This is something that stuck with me. I was the type of person who always did more for my team than I did for myself, and later in life, I found that people who do more when others are counting on them are exactly the type of people that I attract. Through Mrs. Cleveland's influence, I learned **People Will Always Do More for Other People Than They'll Do for Themselves**. To have passion for something, it must matter for more than just yourself.

What stood out to me the most about Mrs. Cleavland was how much she obviously cared about and loved every athlete on the team. She was always encouraging students to come out for track. She was an extraordinary competitive coach, took the sport very seriously, put the highest value on those who put in the extra work to get better and always made each person feel like they were an important part of the team.

To this day, I quote her running tips to my clients and hear her positive voice inside my head. In my fitness community, we discuss personal records and encourage each other to show up and get better. I remind them when they run to pretend like there's a potato chip between their thumb and index finger so that they run loose and keep their hands relaxed. It cannot be held too hard, or it will break, or too soft, or it will fall.

My basketball coach was also somebody I admired. He was an excellent coach and well respected in the community. He nicknamed me Rome after an infamous rebounder that did not have height to his advantage. He believed I could be a massive asset to the team with my rebounding and scrappy efforts on the court. Once again, I made up for what I lacked in experience in effort. Mr. Crandall believed in me and told me I could have a tremendous impact on the team as the leading rebounder.

I still hear his voice inside my head when I need to show up strong, and I relish the lessons he taught us on and off the court. Even though I had other roles on the court, Coach Crandall focused on my strength of jumping high and boxing out. He was a tough coach with high standards and helped us get the most out of our game. Coach Crandall's belief in me became a source of inspiration off the court and helped me to foster a positive mindset and resilience in the face of challenges.

Coach Crandall's influence shows up in the way I coach today. From him, I learned to **Focus on What You Can Do**. If a client comes to me with bad knees and tells me they can't perform certain movement patterns, I remind them of what they can do and encourage them to focus on that. I emphasize the exercises they can do and encourage them to set their mental and physical attention to those movements.

Not all of my experiences with coaches and playing sports were positive. As I mentioned earlier, I played soccer in addition to several other sports. Remember Coach Banana? He was the math teacher I wanted to impress but found very intimidating.

I hate to give this story any energy, but it had a tremendous impact on me in the following years. It was the summer tryouts before my sophomore year of high school. All the players had shown up for what we called two-a-days. During the hot afternoon practice, Coach Banana weighed each prospective team member. He wrote my weight down on the clipboard. He didn't say a word, but after logging the numbers, he looked up from the clipboard with raised brows.

Following the weigh-in, all of the prospective Junior Varsity and Varsity players ran around the perimeter of the soccer field, and the distance covered was measured. I had been training all summer, and I ran hard and strong, finishing with the most laps. Coach huddled up with all of us after the run and said, "I can't believe you let Spraragoni, the fattest girl on the team, beat you. That's pathetic." My last name was Spraragen, and Spraragoni was the nickname he made up for me in ninth-grade math.

The words hit me like a sudden gust of wind. I felt hurt and humiliated and would have given anything to disappear from that field at that moment. I was already overheated and red from my efforts on the run, and I felt like my face was so hot that it was going to burn off. I have no memory of what came after that moment, but that hurtful comment was something I will never forget.

From that moment forward, I thought differently about myself. I had always had a bigger frame and thicker build, and in middle school, I was self-conscious about my height. But by high school, many kids had caught up, and I felt pretty normal. Those hurtful words left a lasting imprint on my self-image. They influenced my clothing choices, my attitude toward exercise, and even played a role in shaping my future career. Three decades later, I cannot share that story without tears and a lump in my throat. I hate that those words had so much power over me, but I believe that the effort I put into changing that negative voice had a powerful influence on who I am today and the story I want to tell.

The influence of my three coaches was profound, as I deeply value being coached and the camaraderie of being on a team. Two of my coaches were uplifting and supportive, constantly encouraging me to push my limits and believe in myself. Their guidance and positive reinforcement were crucial in fostering my growth and confidence. In stark contrast, Coach Banana made me feel self-conscious and inadequate, which was particularly challenging for me to navigate as a teenager. (not sure about this sentence. Feel free to change but doesn't make sense as is). Despite this, combining these experiences shaped me into a more resilient and self-aware individual. These varied experiences have instilled in me a desire to become a coach so I can uplift and inspire others the way my supportive coaches did while also understanding the importance of creating a positive and encouraging environment.

Years later, these early experiences in sports played a big role in shaping who I became as a business owner, a coach, and a mentor to others. I took the positives and the negatives, and I stored them away.

Each experience was built on the one before. Being part of a team in high school led to participating in group exercise, which led to becoming a group fitness instructor, eventually leading to KBC's creation and growth. This is slow, organic growth, the secret sauce to real change and building on your own success. Each of us, through our own experiences, is growing and changing every day.

As we grow and change, we're exposed to so many voices, including positive voices like my high school track and basketball coaches and negative voices like the single line spoken by my soccer coach. All of these voices contribute to who we are and how we grow. But the single most important voice is the voice in your head.

Maybe you already have a strong, positive voice. Maybe your voice isn't very kind to you. Perhaps it tells you you're not enough or compares you to others. Maybe it calls you "the fattest girl on the team."

Changing the voice in your head is possible. Of all the voices, the most powerful voice is your own. When you start cheering for yourself, everything changes. I used to tell my clients who were unhappy about their bodies to look at their favorite things about themselves. Everything changed when they looked in the mirror and focused on that one thing.

Words are powerful. Once you start thinking about the things you like about yourself, more positive things magically appear. Long ago, I learned that nobody responds well to negative coaching. So I don't coach myself in an unproductive way. If you think about the people who have had a positive impact and how they made you feel, you'll recognize that you can create more of those feelings with your own thoughts.

One example in my own life is my Grandma Betty. She thought I had a nice speaking voice and acknowledged me for it. When I have to speak aloud, I always think of Grandma Betty and use it as a positive power.

Fitness is the secret sauce to unlock dreams you might not even know you have. Change the way you treat and value your body, and you'll **Change the Voice in Your Head**. Offer kindness and respect toward your physical self, and you'll find yourself achieving success in all other aspects of your life. Throughout my life, fitness has kept me moving forward. Being part of a team or community and staying active physically has allowed me to be successful in other areas. Sometimes, the voice in your head might say, "You can't do it," or "You're not good enough." But you can change the voice in your head to say, "Yes you can" and "Your best is always good enough."

From a very early age, I adopted the mindset that I was in control of my thoughts and more resilient than most people. I can match my energy to the things that I want to make happen. I don't think I understood what I was doing or how powerful this was until I started reading books about personal growth, business, and leadership as an adult. Using my intuition has been a personal superpower. I let it guide me in times when I felt lost.

"Daring Greatly" by Brene Brown is the best example of a book I have read that speaks to the power of self-belief. Brown emphasizes the importance of self-belief in her work on vulnerability and shame. She suggests that those with a strong sense of self-worth and belief are often more resilient and better able to navigate challenges. Brown argues that cultivating self-compassion and embracing vulnerability are key components of developing a healthy self-belief. Brown encourages individuals to practice empathy, authenticity, and self-compassion to foster a positive sense of self.

While I came into this power of self-belief very independently and naturally through my own personal experiences, not everyone arrived here organically. The good news is that you can develop strong mental strength and powerful self-belief. The research is there. Brown doesn't just say that allowing ourselves to open up, be ourselves, and daring to be vulnerable is the path to living a better life; she also documents an impressive amount of research in all of her work.

You have the power to **Change the Voice In Your Head**. By taking some simple, deliberate steps, you can teach yourself to talk nicely to yourself. You can learn to believe in yourself. To encourage yourself. Then, and only then, can you grow toward your goal. It will happen slowly and organically, but it can happen.

People Will Always Do More for Other People Than They'll Do for Themselves

To have passion for something, it must matter for more than just yourself. Helping other people is a positive motivator. Even if you already want something for yourself, recognizing the benefits to others will always help push you in the right direction.

Focus on What You Can Do

If your knee is injured and you can't do a certain exercise, focus on the exercise you can do.

Hone in on your own gifts. Focus on the things you're naturally good at or have a passion for and do those things.

Change the Voice in Your Head

The single most important voice is the voice in your head. Changing the voice in your head is possible and powerful. Change the way you treat and value your body, and you'll change the voice in your head. Offer kindness and respect toward your physical self, and you'll find yourself achieving success in all other aspects of your life.

Jodi's Story

I joined KBC in 2010 after the birth of my fifth child. At that time, I was severely overweight. I weighed over 200 pounds and had a body fat percentage in the mid-forties. I had all these little kids, and I had no energy. I didn't want to do anything physical and couldn't keep up with them. I had been an athlete, so this was huge for me. I was at a point where I didn't care.

But then, I decided I didn't want to sit on the sidelines and watch my kids grow up and not be involved. I didn't want to be unhealthy anymore; I wanted to be able to live longer for my family. I joined KBC to begin making these changes.

When I first met with Kelly one-on-one, we did a fitness assessment and an InBody. An InBody composition scale is a device that measures body composition using Bioelectrical Impedance Analysis (BIA). It sends low-level electrical currents through the body to assess the amount of body fat, muscle mass, and water distribution. My body fat was 44%. Kelly very matter-of-factly said, "It's just a number, and it will change." Her belief in me was the spark I needed to get started. It was definitely a two-clap moment!

Over the next several years, I lost 70 pounds, and my energy skyrocketed. I remained consistent with my workouts and was motivated by the positivity and encouragement of the community and the changes I saw. During the Saturday bootcamp classes, Kelly often did physical challenges or assessments, such as tracking the number of push-ups or sit-ups we could do in a minute or tracking our time for a mile run. Kelly would give shout-outs and positive affirmations for showing up, working hard, and getting better, even if it were just one rep better. Her encouragement helped push me to keep showing up. I slowly got stronger and faster. With each additional sit-up or push-up I could do, my confidence grew, and I started to believe I could do this.

I began noticing how my workouts with KBC were impacting my everyday life. I had more energy to engage and play with my kids. I could pick up my one-year-old and carry her around or carry a load of laundry up the stairs. I could spend a day at the park and not be completely exhausted. That was everything to me.

On a deeper level, I had a great sense of accomplishment. It felt good to care for myself even though I was homeschooling full time with five small children. One of the regular classes I would take was Kelly's killer cardio class on Tuesday nights. I felt bad leaving the kids with my husband after he had been working all day, but I knew by the end of that hour I would come home and be happy. I would be a better wife, mother, friend, and all the other hats I was wearing. I was better at wearing them because of the self-improvement I was making. I called Tuesday night my "spa night." Gradually, I added more classes to my workout schedule. I felt guilty about being away from my family more, so I made sure to get what I came for by giving 110% to each and every workout. I also started paying more attention to my nutrition. If I was going to be working this hard in my workouts, I needed to be fueling my body with healthy foods and not sabotaging myself with junk food. Change = change!

In 2012, I was injured and couldn't work out. I was crushed. I attended Saturday bootcamp in a boot, and Kelly asked me to help at one of the stations in the circuit. It completely lit me up! I loved being able to help, cheer people on, and still be a part of the workout.

My leadership at KBC developed gradually. As I gained confidence, I began encouraging my classmates, emulating the support I had received from others. I stepped up to be a captain for a Winter Challenge Team, and leading the team became a springboard for me to become an instructor. I was passionate about paying it forward, wanting to support members just as Kelly and others in the KBC community had supported me. Seeing my Winter Challenge team members succeed—whether through weight loss, a change in clothing size, or simply becoming happier—was incredibly satisfying and fulfilling.

Around this time, Kelly had two people helping her during the Saturday bootcamp sessions, Ginger and Brian. Ginger was moving, so Kelly asked if I'd be interested in helping on Saturdays and encouraged me to get certified to become a professional fitness instructor. Once I finished my certification, she gave me a Wednesday morning class at the parking lot where we worked out. I just loved it! I never would have thought I could stand up in front of a group on a microphone and talk through exercises. I felt so happy and satisfied helping people get better. My passion for serving others was playing out in a completely different and unexpected way.

Inergy, KBC's indoor studio, opened in May 2017. Before that, our workouts had been outside in a parking lot. We had a few older clients who were fine with the outdoor workouts, but other potential clients, such as my mother-in-law, were not interested in working out outside on the pavement. After Inergy opened, I thought of starting a small group geared toward people aged fifty-five and over. I approached Kelly, and she was supportive of the concept. Retro Active launched in January 2018 with five participants, most of whom still participate today. I was thrilled to be reaching and helping this new audience. We now have fifteen to twenty people on our roster at any given time. It has been wonderful watching the transformations of our Retro members.

A catchphrase or mantra that keeps me going used to be "You can do anything for a minute," but it has morphed into "You can do hard things." You have what you need to do hard things. A lot of what I do relies on my faith and spirituality, but exercise is very, very similar to that. It's very much a discipline. I use the phrase a lot when coaching people too if there is a hard station or circuit or if they are having trouble just pushing through that last round. You can do hard things!

So many of Kelly's mantras apply outside of KBC, too. Dealing with teenager issues—yes, you can do this. Get out of bed and put your feet on the ground. This is going to be hard, but we're going to do this. We've tackled hard things. We've taken control of your health. It's the same thing. It just translates everywhere, every area of life.

My advice is to stay the course. Make small changes, like swapping white rice for brown rice and chips for bell peppers. It's the little things that matter, but don't do them all at once. Implement one change at a time, allowing them to build on each other. Over time, these small adjustments lead to significant transformations. Now, I eat differently and live differently, all because of these gradual changes. This approach applies to life in general—small, consistent steps lead to profound and lasting improvements.

Kelly's Take

Jodi and I used to attend our children's youth football games together. During one of the games, she expressed her interest in trying bootcamp. I was excited about it and promised to support her. At an end-of-season team party, I followed up with her and learned that she was expecting her fifth child, which meant she would have to delay starting bootcamp. Usually, when people postpone their plans, they never follow through. But Jodi was different. She was determined and true to her word.

In her interview, Jodi shared her struggle with feeling guilty for being away from her children. However, she soon realized that the short time she spent away working on herself made her a better mother and person. Her message is powerful and something we should all note and shout from the rooftops. I particularly appreciate the twist she put on it. If she's going to spend time away from her family to work out, she wants to make it worth it. And she definitely delivered on that promise! That is one of the many reasons I came up with the phrase "Jodi Austin Strong" as a compliment to other students.

During Jodi's first class, I remember her struggling to catch her breath as she moved across the lot. However, her fierce determination was evident in her face, and her goal to be able to play with her children was her driving force. Fast forward fourteen years, and Jodi has become our community's iconic fitness leader. Her invigorating workouts are attended by her children, mother-in-law, husband, and hundreds of other raving fans, a testament to her journey from a beginner to a leader.

Jodi has become a star student, consistently improving her stamina and strength, and she has evolved into a compassionate and vigorous fitness professional and coach. Her unique blend of mathematical, musical, and athletic backgrounds makes her a natural leader in the fitness world. What truly sets her apart is her caring nature and the level of attention she dedicates to every workout, making her clients feel comfortable, appreciated, and seen.

It has always been important to me that my team puts their energy and effort into things that excite them. I perform at my best when passionate and enthusiastic about my work. Our business model allows us to experiment with programming, which is great. When Jodi approached me about starting a specialty program for older adults, my immediate "yes" was a clear indication of my trust and respect for her.

Retro has exceeded expectations and is one of the best things about having Inergy. Participants are incredibly loyal and grateful, and their work goes far beyond general fitness. Students work on brain health, balance, and nutrition. The increases in strength, range of motion, and balance are remarkable. Retro has become its own community within KBC, and they work together to achieve their goals and connect on a social level, which is equally important.

Jodi's Retro program is the perfect example of creating an impact that starts with one person. Jodi had it on her heart to work with older adults because both of her parents struggled with disease and mobility, and she also wanted a safe spot for her mother-in-law to work out. By taking care of herself, Jodi can now help so many others. She has also changed the pattern of being overweight and unhealthy that had been passed down to her. Talk about the ripple effect and changing the voice inside of your head.

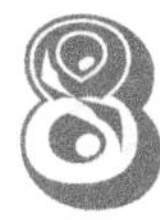

Two Claps

Perched by the small window on an unforgiving chair in the hospital room, I found myself battling both discomfort and emotions. It wasn't just the physical unease but the overwhelming worry for my cousin, Brett, that intensified the discomfort. As I stole glances at my aunt, Maureen, her eyes betrayed the fatigue of sleepless nights, yet they shimmered with an unyielding concern etched deeply within. She remained a steadfast presence by Brett's bedside. This is the same aunt that I would ride home with years later, following my father's funeral.

Maureen's endurance was palpable. She was a portrait of maternal love, drained yet resilient. Her frailty was apparent, and her own well-being seemed secondary to the battle her son was facing. Each passing moment in that room left a permanent mark on me. It was a moment where the fragility of life and the strength of familial bonds came together.

Observing Maureen's unwavering dedication, I realized this was more than a hospital room. It was a transformative experience for me as a young adult. As I witnessed my aunt, one of the strongest people I knew, breaking down, I felt helpless. A determination formed in me. I developed the idea to support parents of sick children in caring for themselves. That was the catalyst that led me to my ultimate calling to help people value their health. This was a moment in time that changed me and altered the course of my life, a seed had been planted, and it was powerful.

As the older cousin, Brett welcomed me into the family fold and made me feel included despite our lack of blood relation. Among the many memorable experiences he orchestrated, one particularly fun event was Christmas caroling. Brett approached this festive tradition with dedication, distributing printouts of lyrics and cheekily urging us to practice, often joking about our supposed lack of discipline.

Despite our initial hesitations, especially at an awkward preteen age when door-to-door singing seemed like a nightmare, Brett's infectious enthusiasm prevailed. We wholeheartedly embraced the holiday tradition. Brett, carrying a jingling can, encouraged homeowners to toss spare change our way—a playful means of earning some extra holiday cash, with us being mere accessories in the process. Despite not sharing in the profits, we sang door-to-door because Brett made it fun. And doing what he said was simply part of what we did as kids. He had that kind of influence.

From a younger cousin's eyes, Brett appeared to be uber-confident and cool. He cared less about what people thought and more about things that were important to him. Brett was charismatic and a strong athlete and student, but he made sure to have lots of fun along the way. He had a way of making any event entertaining with his sense of humor and zest for life. He was somebody I loved being around.

As I went off to college and moved into the next stage of life, he was always one step ahead. In my young eyes, Brett was the epitome of success. He was a Villanova graduate living the dream of a job as a sales engineer in California when doctors told him that they were concerned about his health and suggested he go back to New York for treatment. When I found out Brett had Leukemia, my entire perspective started to change.

Brett's illness hit hard and fast, and he courageously fought for his life, undergoing every last chance treatment imaginable. All the while, he tried to entertain and provide happiness for those surrounding him. One of my favorite examples is the December he was diagnosed when he was probably so scared and upset to spend Christmas in the hospital. Still, he rallied his friends and nurses to dress up as Santa and his reindeer and elves to deliver presents to the sick kids in the hospital. He made the best of a really sad situation.

Amid my cousin's battle with leukemia, he displayed an extraordinary resilience that left a lasting impression on me. Despite his challenges, he could remarkably transform his hospital room into a vibrant gathering place. Instead of succumbing to the isolation of his illness, he reached out to his cousins and friends with cravings for hot and sour soup from the nearby Chinese restaurant.

As we converged in his room, laughter and conversation filled the space, and for a moment, the weight of his illness seemed to lift. Though he never indulged in the soup himself, his gesture brought us together, reminding us of the profound importance of human connection, even in the darkest times. In his simple act of gathering loved ones around him, he reaffirmed the power of community to uplift and support us through life's most challenging moments.

Brett's leukemia could not be stopped, but his spirit, tenacity, and fight left a lasting impression.

Maybe I couldn't help Brett, and the last thing a mom of a dying child can do is think of herself, but I knew I had to do something. I had to find a way to remind people that our health is everything and it's our job as humans to do everything in our power to control what we can. There would always be things that could not be controlled. But I was inspired to take on what I could and to help others do the same.

I knew at that moment that life is a gift. Although we can't predict how long this gift may last, we *can* make choices that enable us to live our best life for as long as possible.

When Brett passed, he gave me power. It came to me when I needed it. I was more confident and decisive than I had ever been. My mission felt so important. Nothing could get in my way. I felt him with me; his confidence and zest for life became my superpower.

My passion became clear when I lost Brett. My passion became motivating people to cherish their health and to incorporate fitness into their lives to feel good. I knew this would bring positive energy into their lives and those around them.

I was a senior in college when Brett died. I immediately recognized this new calling to do something that involved influencing the health and happiness of other people. I had already tapped into the power of fitness and movement for my own physical and mental health.

When I watched Brett battle Leukemia and witnessed firsthand the toll on his mom and our family, I felt like I was being pulled to help others prioritize their health and put effort and energy into the things they could control.

Brett's illness taught me that we all have something coming that we will need to fight. Being healthy and strong was what I believed could prepare us for that battle. But how could I make a difference? How could I contribute to other people's overall health and wellness? I didn't have all the answers, but I knew I had to take the first step.

I would soon be graduating with a Bachelor of Science in Communications. I thought the only way I could effectively help people professionally was to further my education. My new plan was to get my master's degree in nutrition science. There was a great deal of work to be done before I got into a graduate program.

After Brett passed, I knew I needed to act, but I was uncertain what steps to take. I now would have a degree in Communications, which didn't seem like what I really needed. But I took **Two Claps,** and I moved forward. I took the first step.

Two claps is something that I say when I need to move forward. When practicing two claps, I'll learn from everything that just happened and use that lesson to move me forward. I want to clap twice as a restart.

Two claps can also mean "let's go," meaning to do it. Let's just start. Let's just get moving. Let's just take a step forward. Two claps can also mean it doesn't matter. It's OK. Forget about that. It doesn't matter. Start fresh.

I use the expression two claps as a way to not overthink something. If I feel like I'm stuck inside my own head, or I just want to take action, or I screwed up, or something isn't working, I say two claps, and that just redirects me to whatever it is I'm doing.

My students are accustomed to me saying two claps. It's just a way to say, let's go. Let's do this. Come on, let's just do this.

The whole idea of two claps is just don't overthink it. Just brush it off. Go. Just start. Boom. It's very abrupt. They're two fast, hard claps, and it's just like shaking things up.

It's powerful. When we have these mantras that have meaning and significance to us, and we use them often enough and in the right way, they create their own power.

As you've already learned throughout this book, I love to use simple words for phrases to keep myself motivated and in a positive mindset. I always encourage my members to have something that they say to themselves. It can be their own version of two claps.

Get Inside Your Own Head is another thing I say to participants when I'm teaching. I tell them, **"It's You Training You."** You get inside your own head. Even though I'm the instructor calling out the exercises, the voice inside your own head is the most influential. Getting inside your own head means figuring out what you need to tell yourself.

Some other mantras that seem to resonate are **You Got This** and **You Can Do Anything for a Minute**. It's just a short period of time. Just push yourself through it. This mentality works for exercise, but it can definitely apply to other parts of life. A challenging task at work or a season of difficult parenting can seem more manageable if you accept that it won't go on forever. Believing that you can get through it for a literal minute or a season might be all you need to keep moving forward.

A mantra is a collection of words or a phrase designed to free the mind. I encourage you to create your own mantra. Like most things in life, your mantra can evolve and change based on your current season and needs.

To help craft your own mantra, ask yourself these questions:

- What type of motivation do you need? Do you need quick action or to slow down?

- What might you say to a close friend who needed that motivation?
- What words are going to speak to you?

Two Claps

Let's go. Don't overthink it. Come on. Let's just do this.

Get Inside Your Own Head

Figure out what you need to tell yourself. Determine what type of motivation you need in this moment or season.

It's You Training You

Even with an instructor or teacher right in front of you, what you tell yourself is the most influential. You have the power to train yourself.

You Got This

A simple encouragement you can deliver to yourself or someone else that simply means you can do this.

You Can Do Anything for a Minute

It's just a short period of time. Push yourself through it. A literal usage is during a workout when a specific exercise might be performed for one minute. This can be more broadly applied to difficult seasons and tasks. Believing you can get through something for a literal minute or a season might be all you need to keep moving forward.

KK's Story

I've been a part of Kelly's Bootcamp since before day one. I was fortunate to know Kelly before KBC even began when she worked at the other gyms in the area. I was at that first Black Friday Bootcamp on our tennis courts with a small group, mainly her family. And then, the following March, when she started the initial Saturday bootcamp, she did an information meeting at her house, just with a handful of us. And she said, "Do you guys think this would be something you would attend?" And, of course, we all said yes. She started with just the Saturday bootcamp.

After my youngest child was born in December of 2007, my husband and I decided I would stop working. That first year as a stay-at-home mom was figuring it all out and trying to lose baby weight. My workouts were in our basement on an elliptical and treadmill or going to workouts with other friends with babies in strollers. I was a college athlete; I swam in college and swam my whole life. So doing something was always a part of my routine.

So when she did the Black Friday Bootcamp, I supported Kelly and our friend group. And then, when she started the Saturday bootcamp at 7:00 a.m. on Saturdays, I was all in. None of us knew what it would become, but it was pretty simple to commit to.

When I think about what it's become, it makes me a little giddy. It's fun to reminisce about the things that we have done. When the weather was too bad to do our workout outside, we would go to Kelly's basement and sneak down the stairs at 5:45 a.m. so as not to wake up her family. We would move the furniture around and get to it.

During the Winter Challenge, we do a timeline of all the steps KBC has taken. Those of us who have been around from the beginning are like little kids in a candy store talking about everything we have done. I honestly feel very honored to have seen every step of the growth that Kelly and the community have done because many people haven't. Just this morning, at Run Club, I was with somebody who started two weeks ago. On the last run, she wasn't going to run. She's been walking because of some knee issues.

So I said, I'll walk with you on the last one. She started two weeks ago, and of course, she asked me, "How long have you been doing this?" So it's fun to welcome those new people in, but it makes me feel honored to have a front-row seat throughout this amazing community that has fallen into place.

Sometimes, it's hard to explain it to people who aren't part of it. It's more than just having workout buddies; it's a true community. The KBC community goes beyond just the workouts. If people are struggling with something, you can reach out. I'm in a little mini group of maybe twenty of us. We're constantly using each other as resources, like "I need a new dentist for my kid. Does anybody have one to recommend?"

And it's the philanthropy things that we'll do or all the fundraising that Kelly does for the breast cancer workouts and testicular cancer.

It's just such a big part of all of our lives. We're all getting to an age where we're considering moving to a new area in a few years. Luckily, now we have Zoom options because I can't imagine KBC not being a daily part of my life. Before Zoom options were around, our next-door neighbors were KBCers, and they moved to Chicago. One of their most significant things was that they were like, "I don't know what we're going to do. We're going to get out of shape. We're not going to find something like KBC." There are places to work out everywhere, but this little magic goes on when you become a part of this community.

And it's just so much more than fitness. Everybody's doing it to stay healthy and stay in shape. And then with the nutrition components and everything, yes, it's good for you physically and for your well-being, but the mental support, the friends you build in it; it's just hard to imagine not having it in your daily life.

I was diagnosed with breast cancer in June 2015. It was the week of my forty-seventh birthday. It was a shock. There's no breast cancer history in my family. So having support from the KBC community, our neighborhood friend group, and our travel soccer family (all three of my kids play soccer) got me through my chemo. I had sixteen rounds of chemo, then had a double mastectomy. So from June, when I was diagnosed, through the end of December, that's what we went through. But the community was so supportive. On the day of my first chemo treatment, we pulled out of our driveway and around the corner to see a group of amazing friends and neighbors there in Team KK shirts with a big tear-filled send-off.

I was fortunate that I was able to work out through my treatment. I was never nauseous and didn't lose my appetite. Once I figured out my body's response to the chemo, I was back at the lot for my 5:45 a.m. classes with the people I loved dearly. Not only was this good for my soul and sanity, but I know it was great for my boys to see me in my routine. KBC was a fantastic support system to me throughout my journey—and there are some amazing people in my life now because of shared journeys and crossed paths because of this part of my life.

I remember my first workout after I'd lost my hair. I was going to have my hat on my head. I remember texting our friend group, asking them to be there with me. I don't want the people who don't necessarily know me to feel sorry for me. I want to be surrounded by people who know me. And that was all; I'm like, I don't want sympathy. I want to go and get my workout. But I didn't want to be the bald girl with a hat on her head and people feeling sorry for me. And so, throughout my treatment, I was there at the lot.

Since then, I have been a resource for other women (other KBCers diagnosed, friends of friends, or whoever). It's every month, at least, that somebody will either text me or find me at class and say, "Do you mind talking to my friend so-and-so who's been diagnosed?" and they're either going through chemo or having the double mastectomy or looking for doctors. It's being the ear for people, and I'm an open book. There's no part of my story that I will keep to myself. It makes you feel good to be able to listen, at least because it's scary. It sucks. It's not something that anybody wants to face.

Unfortunately, within the past four months, there have been three very active women in the KBC Community who have been diagnosed, which is surreal. But we have our group of those who are currently going through treatment. There's one of them who just had her second round of chemo yesterday—and just being able to be there to answer the questions and to tell them the things they should have in place to help them after their surgery. I am there to answer questions and share practical advice, such as needing zip-ups and button tops because pulling a shirt over your head will be difficult after surgery. I am grateful to help others like people helped me when I was going through it.

Every year in October, KBC hosts an Annual Breast Cancer workout. "Exciting" is probably the wrong word, but it's a celebration. In October, It's pink all over the place. Everything goes pink wherever you look in the world. And some people hate it. My husband hates the color pink because of what we went through. I've always loved the color pink, and I love it even more now because it means something different. For him, it takes him back to that scary part of our family.

I always offered to help Kelly that day. I am not only there as a warrior and one of the ones she's honoring, but I'm also there to help behind the scenes. That's just who I am, and I love to help her with anything. It is such a special day. It's just the feeling of the event. That's the one workout my husband usually goes to. It's just something about seeing that part of the lot decked out in pink with the balloons and the tablecloths and everybody wearing their pink tutus and headbands. But the fact that we honor sixteen to twenty warriors yearly is fantastic. And it's all age groups. I'm fifty-five now, but my journey was eight years ago. You've got all different age groups and nationalities. It's heartwarming. It's just one of those days, and for the rest of the day, you'll just be floating because you know that so many people left feeling fabulous.

I know there are a million other places where people could go to work out. Whether you're working out in a gym or you're doing a CrossFit workout or a bootcamp in whatever town or city you live in, it's being able to get so much more than the workout out of it. It's the connections. It's connecting with the people that you're working out with or the people who are instructing the class. If you go into it with an open mind to get more than the fitness part, you will.

Kelly's Take

Here's another story demonstrating how the tagline "Get What You Came For" can evolve. KK initially wanted to lose her baby weight, but she found a place where she could belong, be supported, and support others. She recommends approaching new experiences with an open mind, which is some of the best advice one could give. KK's openness and willingness to receive love from the community have allowed her to give back to women and families in need during a challenging and emotional time.

As I reread KK's story, I can't help but think that she was ready to start the fight of a lifetime. I believe being strong, fit, and resilient going into her treatment had a significant impact. I also know that they knew they were working with a fighter when she told her doctors and nurses that her goal was to get back to 5:45 a.m. workouts outdoors in the winter. KK has been with KBC since the beginning, even joining the original Black Friday Bootcamp.

Kristen is a role model to me in the way that she fought cancer, the way she chooses to live her life post-cancer, and the many people that she has touched and impacted along the way.

I enjoyed reading her take on the Annual Breast Cancer workout, as it was yet another organic offering from our members. In 2010, shortly after I started the Saturday bootcamp, two students connected to the cause asked if I would host a Saturday bootcamp that would serve as a fundraiser for the Susan G. Komen Walk for the Cure. At the time, I had no personal connection to the cause, but I loved the idea of supporting something that meant a lot to my students. We chose an already scheduled Saturday bootcamp in October to designate as Bootcamp for Breast Cancer. We raised funds with raffles, donations, and guest fees. It was a simple event that started small, but it meant a lot to many of my members because they had friends or family members who had battled or were in the battle themselves.

We set aside a Saturday in October to show our support every year. This event has grown in size and meaning for our community. To prepare for it, Therese (who was also an original member of the KBC Community and now is part of the team and handles the administrative side of the business) will create a shirt design and theme. All our members will be allowed to submit the name of a warrior (past or present) to be printed on the back of the shirt. Most of the work for this extraordinary event is done by the KBC Community. They started stepping up even before I asked, and as a leader, I have learned never to say no when someone has it in their heart to help.

We showcase the stories of our breast cancer warriors through social media and email, one by one. These are women who are currently training at KBC and have been diagnosed with breast cancer. They share how they detected the cancer, their treatment process, what helped them the most during the fight against the disease, and where they are currently on their journey. Their stories often inspire others to get an annual mammogram. These stories offer hope to those who have been newly diagnosed with breast cancer and to those who know someone who has been affected by it.

The workout is different every year, as is the organization we choose to support. One year, a local woman who worked at the deli counter in the grocery store many of us shopped at was diagnosed with breast cancer, so we decided to give our collection directly to her. Another year, we honored a young mom who is no longer with us but had been instrumental in helping our Warriors navigate their diagnoses. We donated the money we raised to Life with Cancer, an organization that held significant meaning to her.

Apart from raising funds and spreading awareness, the goal is to recognize and appreciate our warriors' bravery and courage and express gratitude for sharing their stories and inspiring the whole community. Seeing these women on the other end, with their physical strength and unwavering commitment to their workouts, inspires people.

KK's journey through cancer is only a tiny part of her success story. She is incredibly dedicated and consistent with her workouts, and she has taken herself outside of her comfort zone to sign up for and complete almost all of our nutrition coaching and accountability programs.

She wants to be at the top of her game with her health and energy, and she recognizes that she can better take care of everyone else because she prioritizes herself.

Being on the sidelines of my cousin's fight against leukemia, I experienced the devastation of disease. Over the years, I have seen the impact of my work. I am grateful for people like KK, who have led by example and shown support for those fighting cancer. Sometimes, the path is not direct or obvious, but when it means something to you, you usually find a way to make it happen.

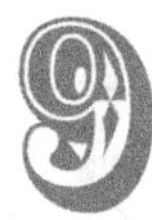

Don't Be Afraid to Fail

In the summer of 1994, I moved to North Carolina with my best friend from high school, Beth. She had been dating my cousin Brett when he passed, and we both were devastated by his death.

During our senior year of college, we began to make a plan in my college house in Ithaca, New York. Beth's college was 30 minutes away and she made a day trip our senior year so we could figure out what was next. We knew that we wanted to be together. It was before the days of searching for colleges on the internet, so we used several big, thick Barron's Books as our guide to finding the perfect graduate school. I would get a North Carolina residency, work, and get into grad school for something in the preventative health space. Beth would get a teaching job and start her graduate work in speech pathology. We both did everything we said we would do and fiercely supported each other every step of the way.

Winston-Salem, North Carolina, seemed worlds away from upstate New York. Our two-bedroom white-walled apartment was brand new. We were on the second floor, overlooking the pool and the tennis courts. We thought we were so cool and lucky to have landed this setup. It will always remain one of my favorite chapters of my life. Beth and I were following our hearts, and we navigated this new world all by ourselves.

I had already landed a waitressing job at Daryl's 1913, a popular southern-style restaurant in the area. During my first shift, I remember standing at the hostess stand talking to the manager, Lisa. In walked this teenager, looking a little hurried and disheveled. Lisa called out as he entered the building, "Oh hey, Andrew. This is Kelly. Would you be willing to train her tonight?"

It was obvious that this idea was not very exciting to him. He had just returned to school after a summer in New Hampshire. Reluctantly, we went to the squirrel (the restaurant's computer system used for servers to check and communicate with the kitchen and bar), and he started teaching me. I had six years of waitressing and bartending behind me, so I was quick to share that I could also teach him a few things.

The bustling restaurant was enormous. It was two stories of tables. We delivered huge plates of food and oversized cocktails to a non-stop rotation of customers. By the middle of that first shift, Andrew was drenched in sweat. He was an incredibly hard worker, helping the other servers with their tables while training and teaching me. The kitchen staff loved him, which is always a good sign.

I went back to my apartment after the training shift. Beth asked me how it was. My response was, "I think the guy who trained me liked me. I'm probably going to marry him."

And so it began—the story of Three's Company. Andrew was our Jack, and we loved having him around. He was three years younger than us, but that didn't matter. Andrew was navigating an undergraduate degree in Finance from Wake Forest while working a handful of shifts at Daryl's restaurant. He was clearly not your average guy.

As my life got busy with community college classes, working part time at a hospital-based fitness center for employees and diabetes patients, and keeping up with my night shifts at Daryl's, Andrew began to show his strong character and thoughtfulness in many ways. I would walk into my shift, disheveled from the day, as he sat at a corner booth with two piles of silverware roll-ups, one for him and one for me. The restaurant policy was that each server had to do 100 silverware roll-ups a shift. Andrew would arrive early so I didn't have to stay late.

One particularly busy night, a single mom in our section lost her pouch (where you kept all of your receipts and cash from the night). It was not uncommon then for people to pay their checks in cash, so this was a substantial amount of money. After the wait staff came together for an extensive search, we realized that somebody must have walked away with all of her payouts and tips from the evening. Andrew quickly reached into his pouch to give her his tips from the night and encouraged the rest of us to do the same. That was the night I took "probably" out of the "marry him" sentence.

Moving to North Carolina right after college and after losing my cousin Brett to Leukemia took guts. Beth and I learned from Brett that life is too short not to take risks and to live life to its fullest. Even from his hospital bed, Brett was a doer. He left us both with the message to stop thinking about it and do it because tomorrow isn't guaranteed.

Beth and I had to be brave to navigate this whole new life. We did it because we put aside the fear of failing. **Don't Be Afraid to Fail** is a mantra I have tried to live by ever since. And I suggest you do the same.

"In Big Magic: Creative Living Beyond Failure," Elizabeth Gilbert says, "You can measure your worth by your dedication to your path, not by your successes or failures." I think it's safe to say that we all have successes and failures. Ultimately, the more we try new things, the more we'll fail. If we continue down the right path, those failures are simply opportunities to grow and learn.

That said, failure can still be scary. But we don't have to be afraid of failure. The best way to overcome the fear of failing is to simply start everything you do very, very small. Then the fear of failing isn't as bad because the failure itself is less intense.

If you're starting a business, don't worry about the logo or the business name. It's all these things that people put so much time into, and then you're going to invest all this time in them. What if it doesn't even work? Just do it with a group of people. Experience it, and then things start to fall into place.

I've attempted numerous things that simply didn't pan out as intended. I didn't dwell on the failures for long. I was also cautious about investing too much time or money into something until I had some reassurance that I was on the right path. Many years ago, long before the start of KBC, I tried to offer an evening workout program at an apartment complex that I lived in by myself after graduate school. I walked around to everybody's mailbox, and I put in a flier I had made. Long story short, nobody came.

At the time, I taught a lot in the mornings. Then I had a day job. Then, at night, I'd have to go to the racquetball court at the apartment complex. Nobody showed up—nobody.

When I look at it now, there are so many things I could have done differently. I could have determined if there was even any interest in a fitness program at that location in that time frame. There are so many things I know now that I didn't know then about launching a fitness program. But I learned something from that experience. I took what I learned from it and moved on. Since I had very little invested (the cost of the flier and my own time), the fear of failure was very minimal.

Later, when I started KBC by offering Saturday bootcamps, I also had little investment. As long as I made enough to pay the babysitter, I considered it a success. Each time I added another class or event, I kept the investment minimal. I wasn't afraid I would fail because the risk was so low. I failed many times. Some of the classes and events were successful and continue to this day. Some failed. I simply learned from the experience and moved on.

If there is something you want to do, a goal you want to reach, but you haven't tried yet, maybe it's because you're afraid you'll fail. Just start it. But start very, very small. Take the smallest, most basic step you can take to get started. Keep the investment very low. If the venture fails, that's OK. Just learn from it and move on.

Don't Be Afraid to Fail

Start everything you do very, very small. Then the fear of failing isn't as bad because the failure itself is less intense. If (really, *when*) you do fail, simply learn from the experience and move on.

Gloria's Story

I have always been a gym girl, dating back to Spa Lady. I was never really into sports, but I could appreciate a good workout. Sixteen years ago, I was a member of a luxury gym in my area, and I attended a class that Kelly taught every week there. I didn't know anybody who went to the gym, but it was fancy and had great amenities. Kelly's class was tough and one of my favorites.

A neighbor invited me to this outdoor workout her friend taught in their neighborhood. I thought, how good could it be? I got there, and I saw Kelly teaching the class. I thought, *Oh yeah, this is going to be awesome.* It was close to home, my friend goes, and it's affordable. I immediately quit the gym, and I joined the outdoor bootcamp.

It felt so different from going to the gym, even though it was the same instructor. I had an instant pack, a gang of people I was a part of. Fifteen years later, many of these people have become my best friends. This group of people started working out on Saturday mornings on a tennis court. We share about our children, know all our highs and lows, and even go on vacations together. That's the difference. She created such an intensely tight community of friends and neighbors.

Some of Kelly's workouts are mind challenges as well. I would show up, and Kelly would honestly do these crazy things, and we'd be like, we got to go. I'm not doing this. This is crazy. But no, we would stick it out and stay and be better off for it. The workouts created a sense of camaraderie, strengthening our bond as a group. The sense of accomplishment led to personal growth we didn't even know was happening.

Kelly would ask us to share your word for the year. Initially, I resisted it. This is dumb. I'll tell you what my word is. My word is "dumb." This is dumb. However, over time, I've started taking it seriously. I've realized that living with intention holds meaning. It's impactful, even if I can't quite put it into words.

Kelly's Take

Gloria's honesty and authentic voice as she shares her journey with KBC made me laugh.

In 2022, she underwent extensive training, becoming a certified yoga professional and joined our team as an instructor.

For fifteen years, Gloria consistently showed up for workouts, fostering new friendships, improving fitness, and being part of a growing community. Even when she questioned things that made her uncomfortable, she kept showing up.

I can relate to Gloria's resistance because I sometimes felt outside of my comfort zone as the group and the expectations expanded. I've always drawn off of the energy of the community, and any of the crazy things that she is referring to were done because that is what I felt people needed. Before planning a Saturday bootcamp, I would think far less about the exercises we would do and more about the feeling I wanted people to have when they finished.

Gloria's resilience in facing uncomfortable situations reflects her commitment to the core value of getting better. It emphasizes that progress lies beyond our comfort zones. As the saying goes, "A comfort zone is a beautiful place, but nothing ever grows there." Gloria's consistency, growth, and gratitude exemplify the beauty of showing up together to get better.

Gloria is a high school teacher at a local public school and uses some of the mantras she learned through the KBC Community to empower her students. She reminds them that "easy doesn't make you better" and that "sometimes you have to keep showing up even when you don't want to."

Just Start

When Beth and I moved to North Carolina and I began pursuing my graduate degree, it might not have seemed like the "right time," but I took it one step at a time. If I had waited for everything to line up, including the finances and the prerequisites, I may have never gone. Instead, I went anyway. I got a job when I got there. I enrolled in the necessary classes to move forward.

In most cases, there never really is a right time. **The Right Time, Which Is Now**, is a way to emphasize that there will never be a block of time or a period in your life where everything makes sense and everything lines up to start. Whatever you want to start, you should just start in whatever form that means. Then you can build upon your own success along the way.

Another example of this concept is that my kids were really young when I started my business. I was dedicated to being a stay-at-home mom. It might not have seemed like the "right time" to start a business. So I started on my own, just on Saturday mornings. I did have to work throughout the week to plan the workouts, meet with all my new people, and manage other aspects of the business. But I could balance that with my responsibilities at home. Then, as my kids started to go to elementary school and they got older, I added weekday classes. When they all got in school, I started adding even more programming.

When my kids were all in middle school and beyond, I opened an indoor studio. But if I hadn't just done something, I wouldn't have been able to take off from where I was. I think I would have waited to start at that point. I would've questioned whether it made sense to start at all.

There are almost always ways to get involved in whatever you want to do that aren't necessarily a full-time commitment. Sometimes, people come to me and say they want to get started into the fitness business. I encourage them to just start training people they know. If they enjoy that, get certified if they're not already. I suggest they start with friends and family. Just start and make sure that they like it. If they start training and teaching, they'll know immediately if it lights them up. And if they feel a connection, they'll find a way for it to consume more of their time. I think this advice works in other industries as well. If you think you want to do something, don't wait for the right time. **Just Start**. We find time to do things that we really want to do. So I think that getting started creates momentum to build upon your own success.

People wait for the perfect time to start something. They think they need to have education or experience or money or a big block of time. Waiting for the right time often backfires. What we find is that as time goes on, you have less of it, and the more you overthink something, the less likely you are to just get started. **The Right Time, Which Is Now,** takes into account that there's never going to be enough time or resources. There may never be a time when it seems easy to start something that's important to you. There's always going to be a sick parent or a child that needs you or other commitments that don't make it the perfect time.

Instead, if you commit to the mindset of just starting and decide to do what you can and let it naturally evolve, then you are much more likely to have the outcome you want. Enjoying the process of whatever you're doing is also really important. The more we think about the outcome as a result, the less likely we are to be successful with something. Sometimes, the outcome isn't even obvious until you start doing it. So if you're too rigid in what you want to do or what you think you should do, then you won't be able to tap into what your work could be meant to do. You have to discover it along the way.

So whatever it is that you're working on, **Just Start**. Whether it's starting a workout routine, learning a new hobby, or changing careers, just put yourself out there and see what happens. Then go from there. There's never going to be a perfect time to dedicate yourself to whatever you're going to do.

In some instances, when you start something even when it's not the "right time," you may face some resistance. I followed my passion and whispers and headed to North Carolina. Before starting a graduate program, my first step was taking the GRE (Graduate Record Examination). This is a standardized test commonly required for admission to graduate schools and business programs. I also had to complete a year's science prerequisites at a community college. Science has always been my worst subject. While being a good student was important to me, it felt like I always had to work harder than everybody else.

In her best-selling book, "Grit: The Power of Passion and Perseverance," Angela Duckworth wrote, "As much as talent counts, effort counts twice." I can relate to this quote in so many aspects of my life, especially when it comes to academics. I've always been able to get good grades in school. While some of that might come from talent, most has come from effort. I've never been afraid to work hard. And most of the time, it pays off.

To get into the graduate program for nutrition science, I needed to have a 3.5 GPA in all prerequisites. I did it. I was on my way. Once I successfully got into graduate school, I felt like I had made it. I came to North Carolina with an ambitious goal, and it was happening.

I loved the food science classes I was taking. I had to fight my way through organic chemistry. And I was finally at the end of the semester for biochemistry. This was by far my most challenging class. I never fully understood much of the material, but I was on track to pass as long as I passed the final.

At the time, I didn't have a clear picture of what my career would look like. A fitness career wasn't what I had in mind. I didn't even know it existed. I had an undergraduate degree in Communications. I still fully intended to use that degree, but I also knew I needed to follow my passion to help others live healthier lives and avoid illness. I was seeking a degree in Nutrition Science because I thought that was a step toward following my passion.

Back to biochemistry class. I can still see the 33.5% in red pen on the top of the biochemistry final exam. The lump in my throat was enormous. It was a two-question test. One of my answers was all wrong, and my professor gave me partial credit for the other.

I fought tears as I stood in line during office hours. While this professor seemed all business in the classroom, the visit proved that he had a much softer side. Through my hyperventilation, he asked me what I wanted to do with my degree. I explained that I wanted to help people be healthy and make good choices with nutrition and exercise. I added that I wanted to be a source of inspiration to those seeking help. He explained that he didn't think I wanted to write diets for people.

As I look back on this meeting with my professor, I know it was a sign, another whisper. It was an opportunity for me to redirect my path but still follow my passion. Instead of making a plan to retake the biochemistry class, my professor helped point me in a better direction.

When you set your mind to something and you're determined to make it happen, **It's Never Over**. Giving up on my mission was never an option. Changing course is not the same as giving up. With the belief that it's never over, you can continue toward your goals even if they look different from what you expected.

I had two choices: Repeat the course and stay on track toward a degree in nutrition science or switch to a new program in which the university had just become accredited. I chose the second option. I would be among the first to graduate from my university with a master's in public health.

Thanks to my biochemistry professor's question, I could clarify my goals and passion and keep moving in the right direction. The next step was obtaining a public health degree instead of nutrition science. However, the outcome was still helping people make healthy choices and being a source of inspiration to those who need help.

Fast forward to my current work; so much of what I do is communicate. While I didn't know it at the time, the knowledge I gained in college and graduate school was preparing me for my future career in fitness.

The Right Time, Which Is Now

There's never going to be a block of time or a period in your life where everything makes sense, and everything lines up to start. Whatever you want to start, you should just start in whatever form that means. Then you can build upon your own success as you go.

Just Start

Don't overthink it. Whatever it is you want to do, just start doing it. Focus less on the outcome and more on the journey. Sometimes, the outcome isn't even obvious. You have to discover it along the way.

It's Never Over

If you set your mind to something and are determined to make it happen, it's never over. Giving up is not an option. Changing course is not the same as giving up.

Rebecca's Story

I joined the KBC workout community in 2015 during the late summer when Kelly offered unlimited classes for a special rate. Initially, I thought it was not for me but only for my super-fit runner friends who joined for the summer. However, I was amazed that one of the girls who joined KBC had a phenomenal body transformation, which she had never experienced while running. This triggered me to want to be a part of this fitness program. I started with one class a week and gradually picked up a second one. By the winter of that year, I was attending almost every day.

Early on, I think I disappointed Kelly. She used to start the sessions with warm-ups where she would talk to everybody and understand their individual goals. She would ask us to share our reasons for joining the class in front of the group to help connect with the students. My goal for that particular season was to get rid of my muffin top. Kelly wanted to believe that everybody joined for some big philosophical moment, but mine was purely because I felt soft around the middle and wanted to change it.

Before joining KBC, running had always been my happy place. However, after incorporating cross training into my routine, I improved my performance in a half marathon by twenty minutes and significantly reduced my body fat. Unfortunately, a doctor later advised me that running was exerting excessive pressure on my knees, and I had to discontinue it. Thankfully, with KBC, I could concentrate on other exercises that helped me stay active while also strengthening the muscles around my joints.

The Winter Challenge has been a big part of my story with KBC. I participated in the first winter I was part of KBC, but the real magic happened when I met my new best friends the following year. We were a group of complete randoms, put on a team with a captain who had never done the Challenge before. Seven years later, we are friends who support each other.

In the Winter Challenge, we talked about the Ripple Effect on the community. My husband was very overweight, and he lost eighty pounds. Although he didn't use KBC, he was inspired by what I was doing and found his own way to get fit. We became more active as a family because we were all healthy and fit. Now, we have two high school boys who run cross country and track, and I don't think our family would have taken that path if we hadn't made the changes we did.

My journey has been about the power of mindset and how setbacks can be opportunities for growth. In addition to my knee issues, I also have lupus and rheumatoid arthritis, which cause me pain and problems with my joints. Doctors told me I couldn't do lunges, squats, or run; I couldn't do anything high impact. However, Kelly and I met and came up with our own set of rules.

Kelly had started saying everything was "figureoutable," and I stopped focusing on what I couldn't do and started looking at what I could do. I can still do mini squats, upper body, and core exercises. I completed adventure races, including biking, rowing, hiking, and even a Spartan Trifecta. Every year, Kelly asks us to choose a word that speaks to our theme and helps us guide our actions and decisions. This year, my word is "bold" because I want to continue challenging myself and growing. Being the best I can be is a big part of who I am now.

Kelly's Take

The stories of students like Rebecca taught me many valuable lessons and are a big part of why I wanted to write this book. Despite not being someone who would sign up for an outdoor bootcamp, Rebecca began her journey before she felt ready, choosing to become the person she wanted to be. Journalist and author Flora Rheta Schreiber once said, "You're never ready for what you have to do. You just do it. That makes you ready." This quote from the book "Sybil" perfectly sums up Rebecca's inspiring journey and the valuable lessons she learned along the way.

Her reason for starting was to achieve a body composition transformation after seeing another runner's results. I recall when Rebecca shared her reason for starting: to get rid of her muffin top. I wasn't disappointed because I believe that any goal you set for yourself should matter to you. I have come to understand that the reason why you started may not always be the same as why you continue, which is a sign of growth. I never wanted people to join my bootcamp just to remain the same.

I have learned a lot from Rebecca, and I hold her in high regard as a professional, spouse, person, athlete, and friend. She has a natural inclination toward growth, being in the right environment, and connecting with inspiring people is vital to her. During our conversation, she mentioned the Winter Challenge and how it has been a significant experience for her. She has been chosen as the Captain's Pick award for her ability to execute and connect on several teams and has stepped up to co-lead the competition for multiple years. Rebecca is a leader with a strong personality, yet she can be an excellent team player in any situation, which is a powerful combination.

Rebecca's husband's weight loss journey and passion for rock climbing did not develop directly from KBC, but they are an essential part of her story. He found something he loved because of her transformation, and Rebecca got emotional as she shared his success. They supported each other even though they pursued different activities. Her husband needed his own thing, and he found it. Now, the entire family benefits from monthly camping, hiking, backpacking, and adventures.

Rebecca's passion and identity revolved around physical activity and adventure. It was inspiring to see how she figured out and found outdoor adventures that were epic, beautiful, and fun. Despite her diagnosis and pain, she remained positive and did everything in her power to control what she could. She invested in KBC nutrition coaching and improved her diet. In fitness, Rebecca learned what she needed to avoid, do less of, and what she could build back in.

It's important to remember that everything is "figureoutable," but you need to have the right mindset, be surrounded by the right people, and have a strong motivation beyond just wanting to lose weight. Rebecca's incredible journey and transformation are entirely her own, but it's an honor to have played a small part in it.

11

Put Your Name on It

After finishing graduate school and earning a master's in public health, I was thrilled to land my first job as a program manager promoting health initiatives for the military and civilians at the Department of Defense in Maryland. While the opportunity was exciting and aligned perfectly with my field of study, a part of me wished I could have found a position closer to Richmond, Virginia, where my long-term boyfriend Andrew lived. We had been dating for four years, and my ultimate goal was to end up in the same city as him.

The job with the Department of Defense was through a contracting company. After a year into the role, they received a new contract with the Inova hospital system in Northern Virginia and offered me the chance to transfer locations to help get that project started. On the one hand, it brought me slightly closer to Andrew. But on the other hand, I knew taking that position would likely delay my ability to move to Richmond to be with him.

The contracting company really wanted me for the Northern Virginia opportunity and said that as long as I could commit to it for six months, they'd love for me to take the lead on getting it off the ground. I would oversee multiple locations and didn't want to miss out on such a career-advancing prospect. Another bonus of moving to Northern Virginia was that my aunt Maureen and uncle Jim lived there with their two daughters, Jaime and Jenna. These were Brett's sisters, whom I helped care for when Brett was sick, and I loved the idea of being around them more.

Shortly after moving to Northern Virginia, Andrew invited me on a work trip and surprised me with a proposal. Living with my family became even more enjoyable as Aunt Maureen and my young cousins were thrilled to help plan the wedding. Maureen excelled at organizing events, and with her and my stepmom Sheila's enthusiasm, planning a New York wedding from Virginia became much easier and more enjoyable for me.

Andrew and I got married. I moved to Richmond, eager to start our life together.

While the priority of beginning my married life in the same town as my husband led me to move from Northern Virginia, securing a job in Richmond proved challenging due to its smaller market, especially in worksite health promotion. Expanding my search to leadership roles in health and fitness didn't yield success. Patience isn't my strong suit, and I was jobless for the first time in my life.

I was optimistic about finding an opportunity in my field, but in the meantime, I was hired by a large health club called American Family to sell health club memberships to prospective clients. I had to work nights and weekends. At first, I was embarrassed that after working so hard to get an advanced degree and experience in the health and wellness field, I would be doing a job that I could have gotten out of high school.

This job did not check any of the boxes I was looking for. My strengths were creating programs, helping people set goals, and coaching mindset, fitness and nutrition. I also enjoyed my experience as a leader in my previous roles.

However, as I was going through the sales training, I realized that I naturally possessed the skills required to connect with people. I realized that I could learn a great deal in a sales position because, other than upselling as a waitress, it was something I knew nothing about. Much of my job would be convincing people who walked in the door (we called them walk-ins) that they needed a workout program. I saw great value in sitting down one-on-one with people. I enjoyed listening to struggles, pain points, past successes, and failures and then helping prospective clients believe that they could be successful this time. After listening to as much as they would share, I would tell them with confidence that I could help them. This was not part of the sale. This was me truly believing in people and wanting to help them find success.

American Family is where I realized that **It's Not What You Do, But Why You Do It**. After just a few one-on-one meetings with potential clients, I appreciated the importance of my role and how the conversations we had in the little cubby-like office could be valuable. When potential members came in to find out pricing and tour the facility, I made personal connections and helped them devise a plan for workouts. My goal has always been to help people adopt healthy habits. Once I sold them a membership, I would follow up about their training and nutrition.

Going into this role, I thought I was overqualified and lowering my standards just so I had a job. I stayed with the company for over five years, and the work that I did made a difference.

Making money had never been what drove me, but I had great success in this commission-based role because I truly cared about the potential client utilizing our services. Because they would succeed at the club, they would refer their friends and family.

I really grew from my experience at American Family. It was a growing, very well-run organization where members and employees were valued and taken care of.

According to Harvard Business Review, if you want to move up in your career, you have to "act, think, and communicate like a leader long before that promotion." Without even realizing it, that's exactly what I did at American Family. The owner, Brian, was incredibly receptive to input. When I suggested that we put more effort into retaining our current members by staying connected and making sure that they were feeling successful, he created a new position and hired a full-time employee in each of his health clubs dedicated specifically to member retention.

Then, to promote the expertise of the fitness staff and encourage the American Family staff to exercise, I pitched a program called Goal for the Gold. We had participants from housekeeping, childcare, front desk, sales, and group exercise. Each individual who wanted to participate was paired with a personal trainer for six weeks. Staff from all departments were assigned a fit pro, and setting goals and adopting healthy habits created a huge buzz in the gym. Members had daily interactions with the front desk, child care, and housekeeping, and the topic of conversation was how much they were benefitting from the one-on-one coaching with their trainer. The entire staff was more connected and energized. The winner was determined by how successfully they worked toward their specific goals. The trainer had to sell their clients' progress to the judges and the winning team was recognized at a red-carpet party with a cash prize from the owner of American Family.

The benefits of Goal for the Gold were numerous, and it was no coincidence that personal training sales were at an all-time high the quarter following the employee health promotion event.

When I was working for American Family, I had no idea that my future would involve leading a team, creating culture and community, or that sales is probably the most important component to running a small business. I learned that sales isn't all bad. If you have good integrity and believe in what you're selling, it's actually fun. I had to be open-minded and it took some confidence to put my own spin on my role. I learned from all the people I worked with, even the General Manager of the club, my boss, who had some values that did not align with my own. Turns out he had a soft side and appreciated the contributions I was adding. The company's owner was very open-minded and receptive to my thoughts, which made me want to be that kind of owner down the road.

I was in my late twenties, and most of my friends from college had professional roles that seemed much more glamorous and sophisticated. That was hard, and I certainly had moments of being embarrassed about what felt like, at the time, a step backward. I had to redirect the voice in my head to acknowledge the opportunity. I stayed true to my standards for trying my best and making the most out of every situation.

Eventually, I was promoted to Assistant General Manager. I would now oversee the fitness director, trainers, group exercise, director of member relations, front desk, child care, kid zone, and housekeeping. I believed in the American Family mission of creating a place for families to work out together, and the vibe and culture of our location had a great reputation.

A new favorite mantra emerged from this experience. Sometimes, you have to **Slow Down to Speed Up**. I thought my goal was to work directly for a company promoting health. But as my story unfolded, I would own my own company. This slowdown was an accelerator to my success as a business owner.

Put Your Name on It is a way of saying, do your best in everything you do. While working at American Family, I owned every one-on-one conversation I had. I brought everything I had into my sales role.

This mantra can be applied in so many different situations. When you show up for a workout, give it your all. Do the best possible job when doing yard work or a home improvement project. When you're cooking a meal for your family, provide them with nutritious and delicious foods.

Putting your name on it doesn't mean the job is done perfectly. But it does mean you take pride in your work. You own it. You make it yours.

Sometimes, you find yourself in a situation that is less than ideal. You can find a way to contribute. You can show up every day and give it your best.

Maybe it's not the most direct path to your goal, but maybe it's the right place to start. **Put your Name on It**. Make it yours. Make a contribution.

At American Family, I never did just the job of my job description. I did my version of my job. I gave everything I had to offer. I did what I wanted my job to be. I used my own skills and made the best contribution I could. I put my name on it.

It's Not What You Do, But Why You Do It

It doesn't matter what your job is. The *why* is so much more important than the *what*.

Put Your Name on It

Make it yours. Own it. Ask yourself how you can do something just a little better so you can feel pride in your work.

Slow Down to Speed Up

Sometimes, you have to do something that feels a little slower. Something that doesn't seem like the perfect way to get you to our goals. But by taking that slower step, you might find yourself speeding up in a new direction. Something unexpected might happen as a result of the slowing down.

Mike's Story

We moved to Northern Virginia from Richmond, Virginia, and I remember telling my wife, Nicole, about this bootcamp I spotted near the Starbucks parking lot. She was looking for a good workout spot, so I suggested she check it out. At first, I thought it was just for women, so I stuck to my gym near work even though I didn't consider my workouts particularly effective. However, as I got to know some of the people joining Nicole, I realized it was for everyone, so I decided to give it a shot about a year later for the 2015 Spring session.

What kept me coming back was the connection it brought to our relationship. Nicole and I rarely attended the same classes but always talked about our experiences afterward. It became a regular part of our family routine. Setting a good example for our kids was important to us. Our son and daughter got into sports, and seeing us prioritize our health rubbed off.

One of the cool things was bringing my ten-year-old son to one of the KBC Annual Breast Cancer Charity workouts. He had a blast, and it showed me how inclusive and fun the whole community was. If I dragged him to the gym with me, it wouldn't have been the same. It's the atmosphere and the people that make it special.

And it's not just about the workouts. It's about friendships, too. Many of the folks we hang out with socially are from the bootcamp. It's like we've built this whole network of friends through it. It's pretty awesome, honestly.

We enjoy the workouts and being part of the community. Whenever I hang out with people in the neighborhood, it's usually guys I've met at bootcamp. It can be challenging at this stage of life to meet new people. Sure, we know our neighbors, but having someone you connect with, especially over the years, makes a difference. Many of the folks we socialize with also attend bootcamp, so meeting awesome people we can socialize with outside definitely keeps me going.

I've always been into sports. Growing up, I spent a lot of time training and on the field. I love the team aspect of the workout and the competition, even if it's just with yourself. Kelly's done a lot to get more guys involved in working out. She noticed that certain warm-ups might turn some guys off, so when she started Dude Camp, it was tailored just for guys. I've made a lot of connections through Dude Camp, even with guys who aren't my age. I'm in my mid-forties, but recently, I played golf with some guys in their sixties who also go to Dude Camp. It's not something I'd normally do, but it's been great.

Kelly's always been great about connecting people and making sure everyone feels comfortable. The friendships I've made are really close. If I needed something and didn't have family around, I could trust this group of people.

Kelly always says, "Put your name on it" during workouts. It's her way of saying, "Own it." It stuck with me. My neighbor and I even joke about it. If he's doing yard work or something, I'll say, "Hey, Rob, put your name on that."

I remember right at the beginning of the pandemic when everything was going crazy. Some people were reacting, while others were responding and innovating right away. Others chose to complain.

Kelly's leadership stood out. I remember driving by and seeing her in the parking lot, all by herself, working out and recording her workout on an iPad for everyone else. It was motivating to see her adapt so quickly.

I thought, "This is unbelievable. We're a week into the pandemic, and she has completely changed her business model for reaching her community." She didn't once say, "Oh my gosh, this is going to be so hard."

It was very motivating for me to see somebody adapt that much and quickly.

Something that has had a bigger impact on me than I expected is Kelly encouraging everyone in the community to pick a word for the year. It's not something I would normally do alone, but it has been helpful.

Kelly wanted everyone to come up with one word for the year—maybe something we wanted to improve or focus on. I wouldn't typically do this kind of thing, but Kelly has a way of motivating people, and I found some meaning in it, too.

She took it further by having us share how our word shows up in our lives during the Friday morning Run Club class. In this class, we do a four-minute run on our own and come back together to do three minutes of strength training as a group. This run-on-your-own, strength-training-together sequence is repeated five times. On the sixth and final run, we all run together, and Kelly has us each share something about our word that week.

Again, this isn't something I'd typically do, sharing personal reflections with a group. But I've been doing it, which helps keep me motivated during the week. Knowing I'll need to share my word on Friday makes me more mindful of working toward it throughout the week.

Kelly's Take

Mike's story resonates with many of the men in our workout community. Initially, he didn't think it was for him, but after seeing the results his wife Nicole got and the friendships she made, he decided to give it a try. It usually takes the guys a few years after their wives join, so he is ahead of the curve. Mike and Nicole fought over certain classes when their kids were younger. It's a perfect example of finding something you love versus just checking a box for exercise.

I can relate to how Mike and Nicole found a new connection through their shared journey with KBC because my husband Andrew and I did the same. The KBC Community provides a space for couples to bond beyond household and parenting duties. I tell all my parents that your kids will benefit from seeing you consistent with an activity of your own, and your relationship will, too, even if you have separate activities.

It's inspiring when our students bring their children to workouts; sharing the positive energy of KBC with younger generations lights me up. The photographer got the most genuinely happy photos of Mike's son Blake at the Breast Cancer workout. It is so important to show our children that exercise can be a fun and happy place. Mike's daughter has also participated in our youth training programs and has been a great role model for other young female athletes.

Many of the men in our classes have sports backgrounds and appreciate the camaraderie of working together toward improvement, similar to being on a sports team. Men are often receptive to coaching and feedback, which accelerates their progress. Having coachable men is one of the many reasons that I value coaching the Dude Camp so much. The guys don't have to be athletic to start; they have to show up with the desire to get better.

Mike's athleticism shines through in competitions, but what stands out is his sportsmanship and supportiveness toward everyone, regardless of ability. The "put your name on it" mantra resonates with him, reflecting his commitment to giving his best in every class. He is the guy you want on your team because of his attitude and ability to make it fun.

I appreciate his perspective on us continuing workouts during the pandemic. I remember seeing his post with a photo of me outside working out with an iPad. Knowing the community was appreciative and receptive to figuring it out fueled me. It is an excellent example of having people around you who support you and can help you to work at a higher level, even during a very stressful period.

One aspect Mike doesn't mention is his role as a coach. He's coached multiple sports teams for his children and has stepped up to coach the varsity girls' lacrosse team at our local high school this year.

His commitment to personal growth and positive leadership is evident in his dedication to youth athletes. Seeing him spreading the values he's learned to the next generation is truly admirable. I love knowing that Mike's work to better himself as a person and an athlete will ripple out to young female athletes.

Jon Gordon, author of "One Word That Will Change Your Life," says, "There's a word meant for you, one word that will change your life when you find it, live it, and share it." For years, I've been encouraging members of the KBC community to pick a word to live by for the year. It's more than a resolution. The word takes on a life of its own, creating meaning and intention for everything you do. But it only works if you commit to your word and revisit your intentions frequently.

During our outdoor workout on Friday morning, participants share how their word is showing up in their lives. Mike is very consistent with this class, especially this season as the head coach of a varsity team. He needs to get his workout in early.

This year, Mike chose the word build. He shared his reason with me in the beginning of 2024. "I want to focus on building a better me, building/enhancing my career, and building a culture of excellence, hard work, and commitment with my new HS lacrosse team (and existing teams)."

It's Got to Mean Something to You

Andrew and I had always envisioned building a life together, and buying our first house in Richmond, Virginia, was a significant step in that journey. This chapter captures the essence of those early days as we navigated careers and embraced the joy of planning our future. Our new home symbolized the culmination of our dreams and the beginning of an exciting new chapter in our lives.

I already told you the story of finding fulfillment in my work during the early years of our marriage. But at home, there was so much more going on. Being a wife and having a family of my own was something I had dreamed of. While I had other aspirations, being a mom had always been my number one goal in life.

Andrew and I are very aligned regarding values and what we want to prioritize in our lives. We come from multiple generations of divorce with conflict, guilt, and negative emotions. We knew that we did not want that in our family.

Andrew's got this analytical, logical mind, while I tend to be more in tune with my emotions and react to the energy around me. But despite our differences, we share a deep appreciation for people, integrity, being identified as hard workers, and nurturing relationships.

Our first son, Dalton, was born in 2001. He fits all the stereotypes of the oldest child. He has always been fiercely protective of his siblings. He sets the standard in our family. Following Dalton's lead, our family helps each other, and we don't leave anybody out.

One early example of Dalton's independence and determination happened when he was just fifteen months old. It was the day I brought his brother Brandon (our second child) home from the hospital. Dalton was upstairs taking a nap, and all of a sudden, his voice seemed closer as he called out for me. He had climbed out of his crib and walked down the stairs all by himself.

Dalton is fiercely competitive. He's both the kid who wants the ball in his hands and the consummate team player. His loyalty, authenticity, and how he walks through life remind me of my dad.

Brandon came into this world in 2002. He pays attention to details and has never needed much to entertain him. He was a very physical child and a natural athlete. Brandon is empathetic, worried about the feelings of other people, and naturally wants to protect them. He's a great judge of character and has a keen sense of how things work and the importance of relationships.

Next came Cameron, born in 2004. He was such an easy child; he went very well with the flow. He loved to eat, had a constant smile, and would laugh at pretty much anything his brothers did. Cameron, a perfect combination of strong and coordinated, also excelled in sport and play. Cameron could get along with everyone and stole the heart of any adult he met.

Once we had three boys, I think we overwhelmed most people. Admittingly, it was a lot. They were very energetic and physical. I may not have done the best job keeping them calm, but they were a trio of fun. The chaos was part of who we had become as a family. My father affectionately called them the "on" brothers. It wasn't just because all three of their names ended in "on," but because they never seemed to switch off.

Three years later, in 2007, Lindsay joined and completed our family. Having a girl was something I always wanted and just couldn't let go of. Andrew was not convinced that we would have a girl the next time, but I knew we would.

We never discovered the sex of any of our children before they were born. When Lindsay arrived, I was the one to announce that we had a girl. My father was the first person I phoned. When I shared the news with him, his voice cracked in response. It was the first time I heard my dad cry. Lindsay was only six months old when my father passed away, and he had only met her once.

As Lindsay grew up, I realized that the girl I was raising was the person I had dreamed of. I had seen her before she was here. I knew that I was meant to have a daughter.

Lindsay is a strong soul who has always known what she wanted and how to get it. As a child, she was demanding because she knew what she wanted. At the same time, she was easy because her wishes were consistent and clear. She has always been nurturing and helpful to younger children and her older brothers and has a unique relationship with each of them. While I see myself in Lindsay, she is very much her own unique person with strengths and traits far beyond my own. Although it is hard sometimes as a mom, my favorite thing about her is her independence.

As all four of my kids grew, we became immersed in their activities and development. We were committed to helping them succeed in whatever they decided to do. I am not sure if this is a good thing or a bad thing, but we never really pushed them to sign up for stuff. If it wasn't their idea, we would not suggest it. Our three boys all chose to play lacrosse in college, and it is a bonus chapter that has been fun to be a part of.

I owe credit to Andrew for calming me down when I'd get stressed about what our kids were or weren't doing. His reassurance was always the same: "They'll figure it out."

My kids were raised with Kelly's Bootcamp being a regular part of their lives. When I taught night classes in the parking lot, I'd bring their scooters along, and they'd hang out with the other kids there.

At one point, they grumbled that everything seemed to revolve around my bootcampers, and they felt like I liked my bootcampers more than I liked them. In hindsight, I believe it was beneficial for them and me to have other people to care and worry about.

One funny story about my boys with a happy ending is their perception that I was a bit annoyed for not keeping junk food around the house. My middle son once told his friend we didn't have a pantry because "my mom doesn't like junk." In reality, we didn't have a pantry simply because it wasn't part of the design of our home.

Similarly, my oldest would complain that none of the kids wanted to eat at our house because they didn't like our bread. As they went off to college, they would send me pictures of their grocery cart filled with protein, fruits, and vegetables. They would even complain that the school food was so unhealthy.

The Ripple Effect is powerful, and it took a while, but I began to witness it in my own family. Working out and being healthy is never just for you. Everyone around benefits from the healthy habits of one person.

In our KBC community, the Ripple Effect reminds us that **Creating Impact Starts with One Person**. We're all wired to help people and to have a positive influence on others. The Ripple Effect allows us to do just that. We help one person. That person helps another, and so on. On the surface, exercise seems self-centered, but it's not. It's the catalyst to help others improve. One person at a time. Taking care of you makes everyone around you better.

The Ripple Effect gets its name from the image of a single pebble dropped into the water, creating a ripple of waves. It's a good reminder that a single action from a single person can reach beyond what is visible to that person.

In our community, the Ripple Effect is that we're all getting more fit because the person beside us is getting more fit. The bar has been raised. The expectations are higher.

We also have the opportunity to witness the Ripple Effect in our homes. We watch our spouses and kids become more fit and make healthy choices. Often, that starts with sports.

All three of my sons were football players. Once they were teenagers, we would no longer plan events or vacations in August. Maybe they could have missed a practice or two, but in our house, we were all in. None of my boys wanted to miss a second of the season. High school football was a big deal, and the program at Champe High School, where they attended, was top-notch thanks to the strong leadership and culture. We had weekly team dinners, where parents actively participated in cooking, serving, and being in the room as the head coach talked about the game plan for the week and gave powerful words of inspiration far beyond football.

At the end of the season, I wanted to ensure all the boys on the team properly expressed their appreciation for the team of coaches and the program. Because I know that written expression can be difficult for high school boys, I texted all the boys a Google Form with specific, easy-to-answer questions: What is one thing the coach taught you? What is your best memory?

The final question was: What advice would you give future Champe High School football players? All the answers were meaningful. The one that stood out to me the most came from my middle son Brandon, **"It's Got to Mean Something to You."** Those words stopped me in my tracks. I knew exactly what he meant. I love to give credit to my then seventeen-year-old son as I share those words repeatedly with my potential, current, and future students.

What Brandon wrote on that Google Form and what we all learn sooner or later, is that what we do has to matter. To be successful, to reach our goals, those goals have to mean something. It has to be personal.

The Ripple Effect

It's the effect our actions have on other people. In the KBC community, we're all getting more fit because the person beside us is getting more fit.

Creating Impact Starts with One Person

We're all wired to help people and have a positive influence on others. The Ripple Effect allows us to do just that. We can help one person. That person helps another, and so on.

> # It's Got to Mean Something to You
>
> To be successful, our goals have to mean something. They must have personal meaning.

Kathy C's Story

In 2008, I joined the original Black Friday Bootcamp, but my story is a little convoluted because I have seven kids, and for several years, I was in and out of the workout program because of births and newborns. Before KBC, I would run, push a stroller, and do DVDs in my family room, but there was no real accountability. After 2011, I became consistent with the 5:45 a.m. outdoor class. It was just a perfect time slot to carve out of my day when nobody needed anything from me. It was just me making myself better. The class's accountability made a huge difference.

At first, it was about getting leaner and losing the baby weight, and then it became about being stronger (because when you run, you don't necessarily focus on the strength portion). And then I found that on days I didn't get to a workout, I was not the mom I wanted to be because I was crabby and constantly trying to find some way to get a workout in and then resentful when I couldn't. It just wasn't conducive to being the best version of myself.

Most of my adult friends are from KBC. This community introduced me to like-minded friends, and the energy from fellow participants became a huge source of joy in my life. Now, the relationships formed at KBC are as vital as the fitness aspect. Working out together most days, you're present in each other's lives. We are cheering for each other in the highs and lows of life.

It's such a range; you've got moms who just had a baby, and you know what they're going through, so maybe you can be something for them. And then you've got the moms ten years ahead of you who have already been through that stage that you're in. And we can all draw on one another's experiences and knowledge base.

Today, it's about longevity and making myself strong enough to do what I do. I'm a furniture refinisher, so I have to lift heavy things. And so it's about being strong enough to do my life and keep me healthy and be here for my kids. My dad died of congestive heart failure, and poor vein health is in my genes. When he passed, that was a big a-ha. That was when I realized that this was not just about me fitting into my shorts; it was about trying to circumvent those genes I've been given and doing what's best for me so that, hopefully, I don't have to have the same fate as him.

Kelly's Take

I could write an entire book about Kathy's journey with KBC. She is iconic in our community for good reason. I knew her as a mom who did everything for her family and nothing for herself before she started coming to classes. At first, she couldn't justify her workouts outside of the home but quickly learned that focusing on her needs made her better at everything.

Kathy is athletically gifted, and movement and competing with herself to get better physically are part of her being. She has been an enormous source of inspiration because of her commitment and ability to train through pregnancy and return time after time stronger and more determined.

What makes me the proudest is knowing that Kathy's fifteen years of commitment to our programs will ultimately benefit her five daughters and two sons. She discovered a way to prioritize and meet all her children's needs while still pursuing her health and fitness goals, and as she describes, she had lots of fun and fulfillment along the way.

I recall sharing Kathy's accomplishments and community leadership on social media to honor her milestone birthday. "Kathy Curtin, a mom of seven, fierce determination, consistent efforts, and kind heart. Kathy is not just an athletic goddess and small business owner but also a superhero who repurposes furniture, bringing old pieces to life. She embodies a work-horse mentality, a caring spirit, and brings a special bright light to our community."

Her mom reached out to me and thanked me, proudly acknowledging the example Kathy was setting for her grandchildren.

As I share Kathy's story, the saying that resonates is, "It has to mean something to you." Kathy emphasizes that her *why* has evolved since she started, acknowledging that it may not be the same as when she began. Nevertheless, it has always been a powerful force driving her journey and inspiring the community.

Perfect Isn't There

My work life and my family life continued to evolve side by side. My job at American Family had unexpectedly become a rewarding career. I was pregnant with my third child and being considered for promotion to General Manager when my husband shared that he had the opportunity to take a new role in his company. It would mean moving our family to Northern Virginia. This is somewhat ironic because I had lived in Northern Virginia five years before and had moved to Richmond so Andrew and I could start our married life living in the same city. I had fallen in love with Richmond, was doing well at American Family, and wasn't really interested in moving to an area known for inflated home prices and horrific traffic.

I loved everything about my current life. The idea of moving with two kids under the age of two and having to switch doctors in the middle of my third pregnancy was not something I was willing to do. My husband agreed to commute to Northern Virginia from Richmond (about two hours on a good day), and then we would move as a family once our third child was born.

We moved to Chantilly, Virginia, in March of 2004. We had three boys, three years old and under, and our five-year-old boxer named Cassius.

Every day, I learn new things from my kids. One thing I've learned is that **You Can't Do It All at Once**. I decided to stay at home with my boys. This new job would prove to be the hardest yet the most rewarding. I planned to take them to the pool and go on other fun daily adventures. If we hadn't moved, I'm not sure I would have ever had this opportunity.

Shonda Rhimes, in her book "The Year of Yes," talks about motherhood this way: "You can quit a job. I can't quit being a mother. I'm a mother forever. Mothers are never off the clock; mothers are never on vacation. Being a mother redefines us, reinvents us, destroys and rebuilds us. Being a mother brings us face to face with ourselves as children, with our mothers as human beings, with our darkest fears of who we really are. Being a mother requires us to get it together or risk messing up another person forever. Being a mother yanks our hearts out of our bodies and attaches them to our tiny humans and sends them out into the world, forever hostages."

Being a parent is a job like no other. As we live out our lives working at jobs, building businesses, getting fit, and developing relationships, our job as a parent overshadows all of it, at least for a season, and maybe forever.

During that summer in 2004, I took my three boys to the pool every day. This is something I had dreamed about doing when I was a working mom. When I decided to stay home and work part time teaching group fitness classes, this dream became reality.

Though I valued my role as a working mom, during this particular phase of life, staying at home with my kids felt like the right choice. I understand many parents face this decision, and I firmly believe there's no one-size-fits-all answer.

While working at American Family, I had the advantage of onsite daycare with an exceptional staff, which eased some of the childcare burden. I often worked unconventional hours, including weekends and nights, so my husband could pitch in and balance our childcare responsibilities. However, this meant our family only had every other weekend together, which wasn't ideal. Despite the imperfect situation, we made the most of it.

Fortunately, American Family had an indoor pool, so on weekends, Andrew would often bring the boys to visit me during my lunch break, allowing us some precious family time. We also enjoyed utilizing the racquetball court, where we could let the boys run around and be rowdy while we shut the door and watched them play.

My enthusiasm and dedication to fitness and being part of an organization remained as strong as ever. However, I started to appreciate that you don't have to do everything at one time. **You Can't Do It All at Once** reminds us that it's all right, and usually necessary, to prioritize differently in different seasons of our lives.

The timing of my move and the birth of my third child prompted me to prioritize my role as a mom for the time being.

Teaching group fitness had always been my side hustle, and immediately after the move, I found a great health club with excellent child care. It was important to continue to share my passion for fitness and to have an activity for myself.

I wanted to not like Northern Virginia because I loved my life in Richmond so much. But it was impossible not to be happy in our great new neighborhood with two toddlers and a baby who were surrounded by potential friends. Being a mom was what I dreamed the most about in life. It was exhausting, overwhelming, and a full-time challenge. I loved everything about it.

As you might be noticing, I've found a way to love what I'm doing during all the different seasons of my life. My life has never been perfect. In fact, **Perfect Isn't There**. You can't wait for perfection. You have to ask yourself how you can make a contribution in whatever you're doing. Ask what is available to you right now.

You Can't Do It All at Once

Prioritize differently in different seasons of your life. There are times when our careers are most important and times when our families need us the most.

Perfect Isn't There

You can't wait for perfect. Instead, ask yourself what is available to you right now. How can you make a contribution?

Kathy M's Story

Kathy: It all started in 2017 when my fitness instructor, Ginger, moved away. I'd been going to her classes for about two years and wasn't sure what to do next. Some of the people from Ginger's classes were KBC members, and they suggested that I give it a try. I planned on just three workouts a week, but I enjoyed it so much that I started attending more classes. I loved it so much that I convinced Ted to join me for the Saturday bootcamps during the summer of 2018.

Ted: That's right, and I'm glad Kathy dragged me along. I really enjoyed the variety of exercises and how Kelly encouraged us to work with new people in small groups. By the end of each class, I'd made new acquaintances. It was a refreshing change from my previous attempts at fitness routines like P90X, which I couldn't motivate myself to stick with long term.

Kathy: What really sets KBC apart is the sense of community Kelly has built. It's more than just a place to work out—it's a true community where we've made friendships beyond fitness. Everyone supports each other, regardless of their fitness level or abilities.

Ted: Absolutely. Kelly has this incredible ability to connect with everyone she meets. She even reaches out when someone's been absent for a while, checking in to see if everything's OK. Her encouragement to prioritize exercise, even with a busy schedule, has been a game-changer for both of us.

Kathy: Kelly's motivational sayings have really stuck with us too. "Get what you came for" and make workouts "the best part of your day." These mantras have pushed us during tough workouts and even influenced how we approach life and work. I've even started using similar positive messages with my PE students.

Ted: For me, the Dude Camp program that Kelly started during the pandemic was a real turning point. The intensity of the workouts and the friendly competition among the guys really appealed to me. It's not just improved my fitness but also expanded my social circle. We've got group chats now and even meet up outside of workouts.

Kathy: One of my most memorable experiences was my first Winter Challenge. The enthusiasm and camaraderie of the group were amazing. Some had been participating for a decade! It really opened my eyes to the power of combining individual and team goals.

Ted: KBC has been there for us during tough times too. When my mom passed away in 2023, the workouts gave me a much-needed outlet to alleviate stress and maintain focus during that difficult period.

Kathy: That's so true. Kelly's personal touch and the way she organizes celebrations for milestones and achievements really make KBC feel like a family.

Ted: Looking back, it's amazing how what started as just a workout has become such an integral part of our lives. We joined for fitness, but we've stayed for the community, support, and personal growth that extends far beyond the gym walls.

Kelly's determination to succeed is pretty incredible. One time, she did a 5:45 am run club on a Friday morning, and it was cold and raining, and four of us showed up. She doesn't change her method of instruction. She teaches you like there's a hundred people there. She could have been in a bad mood seeing, oh, there are only four people here and 20 signed up. But she always brings positive energy. Even when things seem chaotic in her life, she can still block that out, focus on what she's doing, and get the energy that everybody feeds on. She's never afraid of hard work or trying to figure out things to make them better, and she wants us to get the most out of the workout. She will try to give you her best right then and there.

Kathy: Couldn't have said it better myself, Ted. KBC has truly transformed not just our fitness, but our lives as a whole.

Kelly's Take

Ginger Katz's story is an essential part of KBC. It started with the check she handed me for the fundraiser, led to behind-the-scenes work with KBC when I was getting started, and eventually, assisting and subbing Saturday bootcamp. Ginger started her own fitness business, which is another positive thing that came from the KBC community. And when Ginger moved to North Carolina, we got Kathy!

Kathy has an athletic background, is team-minded, and values her exercise time. She shows up very strongly to class, quietly motivating those around her to push harder. It's meaningful that Kathy considers the messaging we try to instill at KBC in her teaching. Having so many school staff as members is one of the things that I am most proud of. Our schedule caters to their hours because we consider them VIPs in our community. As a teacher, Kathy must be lit up, positive, and energetic for her students all day. I love knowing that the mindset and energy she gets from her workouts help her to do that.

Get What You Came For was the original tagline for the Kelly's Bootcamp logo. I asked my students in my classes at both Lifetime and Olympus for suggestions, and they said, you always say, "Get what you came for." At the time, I wasn't conscious of it, but when I went into my coaching mode, I took on a persona and believed that the workout was the most crucial thing in the world. I challenge my students to think about why they are here.

The Winter Challenge seems to come up in many of the stories, and the trend is that the big takeaway is the connection and teamwork more than the results of fitness and body composition. It's another example of people joining or starting for one thing but staying or returning for another. Kathy's interview took place before this year's Challenge, and to no surprise, she stepped up to be a co-captain for her team, The Barbelles (a take on Barbie, "She Can Do Anything"), were the talk of the town and won the team portion of the Challenge. When I suggest the Challenge to rookies, I don't sell the friendships or the weight loss. I tell people that participation will likely create a network of people who will cheer for them throughout their journey with KBC. The Challenge is about cheering for your team and yourself.

I appreciate Ted's open-mindedness, his desire for growth, and his genuine thoughtfulness toward our community. He played a significant role as I created the Dude Camp program and was very supportive of the young man, Alex, to whom we were dedicating our effort. During the Dude Camp Challenge, when Ted stepped up to be a captain, I asked him about his team's shirt color preference. He chose purple because it represents testicular cancer, and that was the disease that shortened Alex's life to twenty-five.

Another challenge I gave the men was to fill out a Bingo board with twenty-five health and fitness-related challenges. I promised to purchase $1,000 worth of equipment for Inergy if they completed all the challenges. Ted took the initiative to send text reminders and encourage guys to finish. Thanks to his efforts, we met our goal of twenty-five guys completing the challenge, and Ted even put together their wish list for equipment.

Ted's statement about enjoying the bootcamp experience because it allowed him to work with people he didn't know demonstrates that he's a strong candidate for KBC. Our program aims to challenge individuals to step out of their comfort zones, and Ted's willingness to embrace this challenge is a positive indicator of his potential success in the program.

I wanted to create a unique atmosphere for Dude Camp, so I adapted the exercises, music, and team-building activities to fit the wants of the dudes. Instead of being an instructor, I take on more of a coaching role as the guys respond better to that approach. Ted is one of our most receptive participants, and he always provides valuable feedback to improve the program and tailor it to the guys' needs and preferences.

I appreciated Ted's compliment about how I show up to class because I'm fully aware of the sacrifices students make to be there and how hard it can be to show up. It's important to me that they receive my best version in every class. Even if the numbers are small, my goal is always to over-deliver to those who show up, especially in the cold and rain!

14

Trust Your Gut

Andrew and I have always had a dog as part of our family. Our first dog, Cassius, became a cherished part of our family in 2000. Cassius endeared himself to us from the start, warmly welcoming each of our four newborns home from the hospital with unwavering protection. He was the kind of dog that turned wary children into raving dog fans. Sadly, Cassius was diagnosed with cancer during the same week my father passed away. Determined to give him the best chance at quality life, we enrolled him in a cancer treatment study. The treatment prolonged his life by eight precious months, allowing us more time to cherish his presence in our family.

Winston joined our family in 2009, quickly earning the title of the gentle giant. We affectionately dubbed him the "regulator" of the neighborhood due to his innate knack for guiding and overseeing both other dogs and our own children. He seemed to have a natural inclination toward protection and leadership, always watching over us with a vigilant eye. His presence brought a sense of cohesion to our family; the kids especially formed a deep bond with him, and he became the cornerstone of our household.

Losing Winston in 2017 hit us hard, especially with my mother's passing just two months later and the opening of Inergy the following month. It was an incredibly tough period, made more challenging because the kids were now old enough to fully comprehend the losses we were facing.

And then along came Reggie. His arrival into our family perfectly epitomizes the philosophy of "Everything Matters." It's a testament to the idea that when you truly desire something, you should put it out into the universe.

We had been trying to adopt a bullmastiff for over a year through two different rescue organizations. We passed home visits, and there were several dogs we expressed interest in. Because we had four kids and lots of people coming in and out of the home, temperament, and history were important.

It had been a year since Winston passed. All four kids were saying the only thing that they wanted for Christmas was a dog like Winston. They still believed in the magic of Santa.

As the family's pleas persisted and adoption seemed unlikely, I reluctantly began researching breeders. I knew it was time for our family to welcome a new dog, but I strongly believed in adopting a dog needing a home.

The next morning, as I enjoyed my pre-workout coffee and flipped through the newspaper, a powerful image grabbed my attention: a pound in Florida captured in a large color photograph. Striking large-breed dogs were tethered to the fence outside the pound, an overflow caused by owners leaving their pets behind instead of making boarding arrangements. This poignant image left a lasting impression on me, almost like a sign. It was just before Thanksgiving, and the caption beneath the picture emphasized the heartbreaking truth: "Dog owners abandon pets so they can go on vacation."

As you already know, I believe in signs and have learned to take action when I get them. The whispers we hear and the feelings we get—they all mean something. The only way we can find out what they mean is to act on them.

On the day when I came across the picture of chained dogs in Florida while teaching my morning outdoor bootcamp at 5:45 a.m., I shared with my students the story of my family's request for a bullmastiff. During the class, I mentioned that I was contemplating purchasing one from a breeder and how the image of dogs needing homes served as a timely reminder that there were dogs out there needing homes.

When I got home that morning, I received a text from Candice, one of my students who was in class that day. Candice said her cousin and his wife live in south Florida, and they breed and show bullmastiffs. They are very connected to the bullmastiff rescue world. Candice (also a mom of four) offered to contact them on my behalf. The cousin connected me to a woman named Lindy from Pittsburgh. As soon as we were connected with Lindy, I knew we were on the right path. Sometimes, you have to trust your gut and believe in the power of intuition.

Trusting your gut is really just another way to say you have confidence in yourself. It's important to follow your own intuition. Most of the time, we know what our next step should be. We might just be afraid to take it. But trusting your own gut, your own intuition, is powerful.

Lindy, a true animal lover, philanthropist, and kind soul, put me through the wringer. We had multiple conversations for at least a month. There were lots of questionnaires and conference calls with Andrew and her husband Vince.

After multiple conversations over the next month, Lindy said she would drive to our home with eight-month-old Ace (who we renamed Reggie) on December 26 to see if we were a good fit. I felt I had landed the most important job of my life.

Because I had so many conversations with Lindy, I felt such a connection to her. She was very detail-oriented and wanted to be sure we were properly educated and prepared for this adoption. We were all blown away that she drove Ace from Pittsburgh with blankets, toys, supplements, and food. She was clearly very attached to Ace, but she knew that he needed a family of his own. She was crying when she left our home. What a lesson and a gift we received.

This whole experience was significant on so many levels. The picture I saw while drinking my coffee mattered. Each person and their actions mattered. All of these things together led to Reggie joining our family.

Reggie was the greatest gift the six of us have ever received. He has been a constant source of comfort and joy. He was born on St. Patrick's Day and nicknamed a leprechaun, which makes sense. He magically brings us all together as a family. Having Reggie during the pandemic was a blessing that none of us could have predicted.

In the book "Signs: The Secret Language of the Universe" by Laura Lynn Jackson, we're told that "people cross our paths and enter our lives as either a blessing or a lesson. Often, it is both. Either they have something to teach us, or we have something to teach them, or, at best, we have something to teach each other. That is how this great chain of light and interconnection works."

When KBC is together as a community, **It's More Than a Workout**. Crossing paths with each other during a workout is a blessing and sometimes a lesson. We come together to help each other and to be helped. We come together to teach one another and to learn from one another.

Trust Your Gut

Practice tuning into your intuition regularly. Start by paying attention to the subtle feelings, thoughts, or sensations that arise when making decisions. Trust your instincts in small matters and observe the outcomes. Over time, as you become more attuned to your inner voice, gradually apply this trust to larger decisions and life choices.

Listen to the whispers and watch for the signs. Then, trust your own thoughts and feelings. Take action.

The Power of Intuition

Most of the time, we know what the next step should be. We might just be afraid to take it. Trusting your own intuition is powerful. Having confidence in yourself and believing that your intuition is right will lead you down the right path.

It's More Than a Workout

Crossing paths with each other during a workout is a blessing and sometimes a lesson. We come together to help each other and to be helped. We come together to teach one another and to learn.

Julie's Story

I used to work out and coach at South Riding CrossFit in the same shopping center as Inergy. However, I had to stop due to a severe injury. I herniated my disc and had two bulging discs in my back. As a result, it became challenging for me to engage in high-intensity activities such as explosive workouts and deadlifting.

I began exploring more strength programs and eventually shifted away from CrossFit. I created my own program and continued doing strength exercises during CrossFit's open gym hours. As people began to notice my progress, they started asking me about my routine. I explained what I was doing, and the CrossFit gym owner agreed to let me run a strength program for members interested in building their strength without focusing on CrossFit. The program was well-received and popular among female members, but unfortunately, the gym eventually closed down. Despite this setback, I remained committed to teaching strength training and believe that it is vital for people to maintain their strength as they age.

I'm a dietician by trade. I have worked in hospitals and home care and have seen how the older population can become deconditioned. They often require assistance with simple daily activities like getting off the couch or toilet or reaching up to grab something. It's not just about looking strong or toned but about being functional and healthy enough to perform tasks like lifting heavy boxes or picking up a child.

Around the time when Inergy was opening up, I contacted Kelly and offered to conduct strength classes for her community. I shared details about my classes, and Kelly was very interested. She mentioned they had nothing similar in their programming and thought her people would love it. I started teaching twice a week in the evenings.

The KBC community is incredibly loyal. They have a buy-in that I've never seen before, and it's a testament to the kind of community Kelly has fostered. She has expressed concern about new gyms and studios opening up and competition from larger brands, but I don't think she has anything to worry about. People are there for community and friendship as much as the workout.

I've noticed that many new people are joining our fitness class. When I ask them how they learned about KBC, they often say someone recommended it. Many seem to be taking a leap into fitness for the first time and trusting the instructors. A respected fitness studio like Inergy can motivate individuals to exercise and find inspiration, and I enjoy welcoming new lifters and making them feel comfortable.

When I reflect on our community, the word that immediately comes to mind is "supportive." It's truly remarkable to witness how individuals come together to motivate and encourage one another, whether it's during birthday pushups or in my strength class. They cheer each other on, saying things like "You've got this!" and "Just one more!"

Many people who attend my class have never worked with a barbell or done any lifting before. They realize that stepping out of their comfort zone and getting comfortable with being uncomfortable is necessary to succeed. This helps them gain confidence in the gym and outside it. They feel empowered to lift heavy boxes or their grandkids using the proper mechanics without injuring themselves. The trust they gain during class carries over to their daily activities, making them more functional and independent.

Teaching at Inergy has been a very positive experience. I enjoy being part of the supportive community and getting to know the members and their families. Kelly trusts me to teach important but not commonly taught things, which is rewarding.

Kelly's Take

Ironically, when I wanted to rent the space that Inergy is currently occupying, the management company hesitated because they thought I would directly compete with CrossFit. I explained that I had already been running my business one mile away for eight years, and the owner and I had a good relationship, as we served two different markets.

While Inergy was designed to complement outdoor programming and add variety, I intentionally avoided CrossFit-style workouts out of respect for them.

When Julie said she wanted to start a strength program to teach proper lifting techniques and introduce strength training, I felt like I was dreaming. I wanted Inergy to maximize offerings to our current students and attract new ones. Julie had an incredible reputation and credentials, and I liked her style, which was very different from mine. Despite my tenure in the fitness space, I never really spent time in the weight room and leaned on Julie's expertise. Julie is why we have so many plates and barbells in the studio. She told me exactly what to get, and the equipment she had selected has been incredibly well utilized since the summer of 2017.

Our members love Julie and her classes, and her programs sell out. She is earnest about what she does (which I love), and her desire to make others feel comfortable and competent with lifting makes her very approachable. As she mentioned, she introduced many people with no prior lifting experience to weight training.

Julie was the first person I hired who was not part of the workout community beforehand. It was more of a partnership because she had already developed a successful program.

One important saying I often have to remember is to stay in your lane. There's so much about the health and fitness space that I value. Opening Inergy connected me to some professionals who had skill sets beyond my own. The amount of trust and respect I had for Julie came from my gut. As I've shared throughout this book: Your gut is usually right.

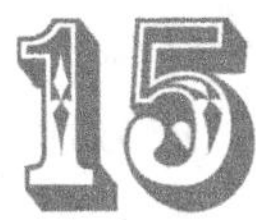

Pick One Thing, Nail It,
Then Add On

When I heard the whisper on the way home from my dad's funeral and the strong calling to follow my passion during the Black Friday Bootcamp in 2008, I had no idea how things would unfold.

I followed my instincts and started offering a once-per-week bootcamp workout. I found outdoor space and began spreading the word that I was starting a workout program where attendees could expect to challenge themselves physically and mentally. Word-of-mouth promotion quickly ensued as interested participants eagerly shared the news with their neighbors and friends. After all, trying something new and different is always more fun with friends by your side.

A few weeks before the first workout, I hosted a meeting at my home for those who had signed up. During the meeting, I laid down some expectations and shared my three goals for the program. The rule was that if you were in town, healthy, and if a child who depends on you did not require immediate attention during the hour, you were expected to attend. Otherwise, I expected you to inform me beforehand via email. I also told them that even though it was only a once-a-week workout, I wanted to treat it as a program where they would be given some homework throughout the week. I demonstrated some body weight exercises we would be doing in my family room. I encouraged everyone to schedule a one-on-one appointment so I could assess where they were starting and help with some short-term goal setting.

My objectives for the program, when I started, are still written on my website today with the exact wording that I shared that night:

1. Get people to exercise (especially those who wouldn't otherwise).

2. Make it affordable.

3. Require accountability.

4. Have fun.

During my Saturday morning bootcamps, I devised various ways to keep the participants engaged and motivated. I incorporated games, partner exercises, challenges, and circuits to add variety and excitement. As a coach, my style is to focus on the positive aspects of each individual, encouraging them to achieve their goals. One specific aspect of my coaching style is that I cheer for people. I noticed my students quickly picked up on this and began doing the same. To help my students see their progress, I offered assessments where they could track growth in reps per minute, the timed mile, and signature workouts where they would record their scores.

I needed a better system for signing up people and taking payments. However, I managed to collect emails through registration forms and started building an email database. I would send weekly motivational messages that included shout-outs for students who had excellent attendance, achieved a personal record, or showed strong leadership skills. I enjoyed recognizing my students for their hard work and accomplishments, and these emails were a way for them to get to know each other.

I also shared homework, shout-outs, and inspiration throughout the week.

On a Saturday morning, right after I finished my bootcamp, I received a flurry of text messages from members of Olympus Gym. They informed me that the owners had emptied the gym in the middle of the night without prior notice, and now the doors were locked. The situation worried many of my bootcampers, who were also students at Olympus. They were concerned about my equipment left at the gym and the weekday classes we used to do together.

However, this unfortunate event turned into an opportunity for my business to grow organically. I assured my students that they didn't need to worry and that I would continue to offer the classes I taught at Olympus but at our outdoor location instead. Surprisingly, the program gained momentum, and I eventually added morning classes throughout the workweek.

I sought the help of bootcamp participants to form a team of instructors. Working together, we have expanded our reach, services, and offerings. Our program now includes:

- Comprehensive nutrition coaching
- Small group training options
- Accountability coaching
- An indoor training studio called Inergy

In addition, we implemented cutting-edge virtual training technology. Our team is passionate about helping people lead healthier and happier lives, and we take pride in what we do.

I took a path that was risky and without much direction. I didn't have a business plan, a niche market, or any sense of where I wanted to go. What I did have was an overall mission to promote health and prevent sickness. My passion and purpose guided my every move.

In building all this, I followed a strategy of **Pick One Thing, Nail It, Then Add On**. This is a strategy that works for most goals, and it leads to success and minimizes the risk of failure. I ensured our Saturday bootcamp program was strong before offering weekday classes. I became proficient at leading large group classes myself. Then I started to bring other team members into the mix. Our outdoor program was successful and stable, so I opened an indoor studio.

It's essential to take a gradual approach when improving your fitness level. Rather than trying to do everything at once, consider starting with a small, manageable change. For example, if you're not currently exercising at all, you might begin by adding a few walks to your routine each week. This can help you build momentum and get into the habit of being more active. Once walking is a regular part of your routine, you can add other types of exercise, such as strength training or group fitness classes. This gradual approach can help you avoid feeling overwhelmed or burned out and can ultimately lead to sustainable, long-term results.

It's worth noting that I didn't achieve this alone. My team of talented instructors, affectionately known as The Dream Team, played a crucial role in making it happen. It all began with asking one person for help. In 2010, I only offered outdoor bootcamps, and the classes had grown significantly, making it difficult to keep up with everyone. When thinking about who could assist me, I remembered my children's physical education teacher. He had impressed us with his exceptional and innovative field days. He also had a friendly personality and knew all the children personally. My sons idolized him. He became part of my Saturday bootcamp team until his kids reached the age where they had their activities.

I also asked Jodi and Ginger for help because they were already stepping up and were natural leaders within the group. They would assist me in setting up equipment and coaching the participants through stations and circuits. With their assistance, we could divide the students, create competitions, and expand our capabilities. Having additional support on Saturdays made the classes even more special.

We spent the first eight years of our business conducting all our workouts exclusively outdoors, regardless of the extreme weather conditions. Since we didn't have an indoor option, we became known as the "crazy people" who trained in the snow and rain all year round. We only moved our sessions indoors to my oversized garage during single-digit temperatures or electrical storms. We still identified ourselves as an all-season outdoor bootcamp and felt unstoppable. In the winter of my seventh year in business, several people approached me within a short period of time, asking me to consider opening an indoor training space. They cited medical reasons that prevented them from working out in the cold and the fact that the pavement was too hard on their joints. They made it clear that they genuinely miss working out with the community. That part tore at my emotions.

I had some concerns about opening a studio, and the biggest one was protecting my passion. I loved pulling up my fully stocked van to a parking lot, unloading the equipment, and teaching my class. I did not have to pay rent or manage a facility or a team. All my energy could be spent coaching and helping people willing to work out in a parking lot achieve fitness goals far beyond anything they ever could have imagined.

Another issue I faced was the high rental price in the desired area I had wanted to operate out of. I had calculated the numbers and concluded that it would be difficult to accommodate the number of people I had on Saturday mornings with such rental prices. I required a spacious area with ample parking space, but finding such a place within my budget seemed impossible. So I contacted a well-connected broker who understood my requirements and budget constraints. Unfortunately, he too agreed that finding a suitable space was impossible.

This was the moment when I started thinking differently. I realized I didn't have to move my Saturday bootcamp inside. Instead, I could continue to operate my outdoor offerings, including the Saturday bootcamp, in the parking lot while also opening up a studio to offer a broader range of services to our existing members and potential new ones.

Before I found an affordable indoor space, I wanted to see if people would pay a little more to work out with a smaller group. Until then, I had been leading all of my classes in a local parking lot with very little overhead and large classes. However, to run an indoor studio, I needed people to invest a little more. So I enlisted the help of Erica and Jodi to help me start a small group training program, which we named Camp U.

Amy, whose story is shared in detail in Chapter 2, was already coaching nutrition, and her camp would include a nutrition and fitness component.

Also, Jess and Jenny started teaching barre in my garage during this time. Both were star students with dance backgrounds. Barre exercises often involve small, controlled movements performed in repetitions, suitable for all levels. These classes were different from the bootcamp-style class I had been offering until now, which was exactly what

I wanted. We didn't have an indoor studio yet, but I wanted to gauge interest in different kinds of classes and build a schedule of classes.

In 2017, when we opened the indoor studio, I built a team of six people. All six of these instructors were already members of the KBC community. They were all regular participants in Saturday bootcamp, and a few of them had been team captains in the Winter Challenge, a very involved program offered by KBC to build community and increase overall fitness.

When building a team, I didn't seek out local people who were already instructors. Instead, I looked for members of our own community who I believed had the capacity and skill to become instructors. Then, I helped them take the proper steps to become instructors. I guided them in getting certified and obtaining other industry education. Most importantly, I allowed them to practice teaching right in our community, and I believed they would each develop into dynamic instructors.

Eventually, I hired some outside instructors who did a beautiful job of bringing something unique to the community. They have offered distinct classes that would not otherwise be available to our community.

The growth of the KBC Dream Team is yet another example of **Slow Organic Growth**. Each of these instructors has their own unique journey of becoming a leader within the community. One change led to another that led to another. A growing number of participants on Saturdays led to hiring assistants during those class times. The idea of opening an indoor studio led to the development of a small group training program and the offering of other styles of fitness, like barre and yoga. And we're not finished with this growth yet. I just hired a brand-new instructor. And she's the daughter of one of our original bootcampers. I can't wait to see what she brings to the KBC Community.

The most direct path to success comes through taking steps. You don't do all these things at once. You create one habit. You do it so much that you finally recognize that you don't even have to think about that anymore. Then, you work to create another change.

Many of my bootcampers will tell me, "Kelly, I got the workouts. There's zero chance I'm not working out." Working out has become part of who they are. That's how they know it's time to consider other aspects of their health. It's time to focus on other things that might benefit their overall wellness. Some next steps might be water tracking, getting more sleep, or meditating.

The people who have been with me the longest have certain habits that they're just competent in. They're just who they are, but they're not content. They're still trying to make a change, to make improvements. They're still trying to get better. So they're taking other things and challenging themselves in other ways.

Change = Change is another mantra to illustrate this type of progress. Start with one change. Do it well. Do it until it becomes second nature. Then work on the next thing. For example, start by making exercise a habit. Then, once exercise is regularly done, start working on another health concept. Maybe it's better nutrition. Maybe it's more sleep.

This model is explained well in James Clear's book, "Atomic Habits." Clear states, "Success is the product of daily habits, not once-in-a-lifetime transformations." What we do daily and our habits lead to real change.

Slow organic growth takes time, but the successes lead to sustainable change.

Pick One Thing, Nail It, Then Add On

The most direct path to success has steps. You're not trying to do all these things at once. You create one habit. You do it so much that you finally recognize that you don't even have to think about that anymore. Then, you work to create another change.

Slow Organic Growth

Growth that happens naturally, without being forced or coerced, often happens slower. Organic growth can still be intentional but involves observing what's already happening and determining what is needed next.

Change = Change

Start with one change. Do it well. Do it until it becomes second nature. Then work on the next thing. For example, start by making exercise a habit. Then, once exercise is regularly done, start working on another health concept. Maybe it's better nutrition. Maybe it's more sleep.

Mo's Story

I started with KBC in 2011. I was reluctant to try it because I felt it was a program designed for women, but my wife was sure I would like it. The last time I had significant exercise was in the army. My buddies and I would go to the gym after work and lift. I have always considered exercise in terms of physical accomplishment; benefits like weight loss might happen, but it wasn't the goal. I struggled to find the right place to work out and was pretty pessimistic when I started.

From the first class, I knew it was the real deal. I started with Saturdays and slowly ticked up to at least five to six times a week. KBC has affected our decision to stay in this area. I'm more of a city guy, but this community has come to mean something to me, and I think more about long-term health. This is a change in my thinking.

I showed up for the first workout and was out of breath in the warm-up. I tried not to get too wrapped up in the fact that I couldn't keep up, just focusing on what I could do. Not getting discouraged made me get ahead, increase the weight I lifted, move faster, and get stronger.

We all need to be healthy mentally and physically. KBC provides that balance by using fitness to help regulate other life issues, like stress. Knowing you can go to a workout after a tough day and look forward to it is powerful.

Kelly likes to try to get our buy-in when she's starting something new, and when she was thinking about Dude Camp (a program designed exclusively for men), she met with some of the guys about the idea. I was skeptical; what's the difference? We all show up anyway. It's going to be the same dudes. Turns out it was a really good idea to attract new guys (who might have shared my original mindset of group fitness being for ladies) to the program. I think for other guys, it's a sense of camaraderie. They feel comfortable in this environment, and it's guys supporting guys.

Kelly's Take

Mo is my ideal client who is honest and authentic. I can best serve people like Mo because I value that I had to earn his respect as a coach and a trainer. I feel similar to him in that I have to experience something firsthand to know if it's a fit for me, and I liked the challenge of convincing him that our workouts are the real deal.

Mo is very complimentary of the workouts and the programs, which means a great deal because he backs it up with his effort and commitment. I know it bothered him at first; I was in better shape than him, and I distinctly remember the morning, just a short time after he started, that we were running hills, and he passed me on the right. Game on, Mo. I tease him that he's grumpy and a man of few words, but it has great value when he shares. He thinks and cares about other people, which is just one reason that the community aspect of KBC is important to him.

Because of his intense ability to push himself physically, he quickly became an icon in the community. Mo was no-nonsense and not here for the small talk when he started. With consistency and determination, he has become one of our community's strongest and most fit men. If he's your partner for a workout, you are guaranteed to be motivated and pushed. He genuinely cheers for others, has stepped up to make others feel welcome, and has contributed to the Dude Camp Community as a leader.

His inspiring transformation over the years has been the mental part. KBC means something to him; it's where he relieves stress and connects with like-minded people. When working on activities outside of KBC, like meditation and daily movement, he shares them with the community for accountability.

The part of Mo's story that connects with the message I want to share is that just because you came for one thing doesn't mean that's why you stay. Mo's mindset has changed as much as the weight he lifts has increased (from fifteen to fifty pounds). He was not looking for a community or a place to grow beyond his fitness level. Still, by slowly leaning into some mindset coaching and community building, KBC has become a part of his identity, so much so that he doesn't want to move too far away.

Change equals change is one of my favorite sayings. It means different things, but in Mo's case, it's about thinking differently as you evolve.

Therese's Story

I used to be a member of LifeTime Fitness in Centreville, Virginia. One day, a woman was walking in front of me with her children—three little boys and a baby girl. The boys looked similar in age to my two older boys, and my youngest son was a few months older than her daughter. As I followed behind her, I thought to myself, if I'm blessed enough to have a fourth child, I now have a pretty good picture of my life. Well, my life turned out to be more of the same—another boy!

To my surprise, the class I attended that day was being taught by the woman I had been walking behind. She was not only a mom to three young boys and a baby girl but also a fitness instructor. I clearly remember that during one part of the class, while we were holding a plank, the instructor hopped off the stage onto the floor and walked between us, asking why we were there and what we got up in the morning to do. She had an elevated tone to her voice, kind of similar to a drill sergeant, and said for us to get those butts down!

I'm thinking to myself, "Oh my gosh, OK. Really? Who is this person?" Most instructors at the time would just teach, speak some pleasantries, and then leave once class was over. This was a fitness class first, but I was pretty sure taking another one of these instructor classes was my last.

Fast forward several months, and one of my good friends was attending classes at Olympus Gym. She would rave about a particular class and instructor. She had mentioned that this instructor was getting ready to start a local bootcamp class on Saturdays in a neighborhood adjacent to ours. This sounded ideal and would allow me more time on Saturday mornings without having to drive back and forth to the gym. Come to find out that the bootcamp was being hosted by none other than the woman I walked behind at Lifetime and the instructor who told me to get my butt down—Kelly Young! I decided to give Kelly a second chance, and with the convenience and cost of the bootcamp, it was really a no-brainer!

When my good friend and workout partner got pregnant and stopped coming to Saturday bootcamp and other classes, I decided to continue as I had started to establish a great routine. I really enjoyed the workouts, and as Kelly added more classes, I decided to leave LifeTime Fitness. What initially started on a small clubhouse field moved to the tennis courts, the basketball court, inside the clubhouse, an empty lot near Harris Teeter Grocery Store, and eventually to an indoor space with continued outdoor classes and the Saturday bootcamp. It was a new and different experience for me to work out outside, but the workouts were fun with great music, and again, the convenience of what she started to establish was ideal.

I don't think Kelly ever put two and two together that I once attended a class of hers or that I was the mom of the boys her boys had played with at the gym and who attended the same soccer and basketball camps over the summer. I'm more on the introverted side and never formally introduced myself to Kelly. She pronounced and spelled my name wrong for several years before even realizing it. So when Kelly offered the first Winter Challenge and asked us to fill out a piece of paper with the name of the individual(s) we'd like to participate with,

I was a little nervous. I indicated I'd like to be with a mom who had children in the same elementary school as I did and a mom who was involved in the same soccer league my oldest played for. Kelly performed magic and ended up putting me on team with those two moms and two others that were in similar stages of life. We clicked at our first meeting, and the rest is Winter Challenge history, especially considering I discovered I was pregnant with my fourth just weeks after the challenge started. I continued participating in the challenge, and Kelly removed me from the weight loss/body fat component. We ended up winning that first year, and it was a huge accomplishment for our team. Still it proved to be a pivotal moment for Kelly and her vision of what she wanted the winter challenge program to be—a community of like minded individuals who would come together and show up for one another with a common goal.

As Kelly's program grew, I would do little things here and there to help out where and when I could. One day, in speaking with a friend, I mentioned that I'd like to try and find a little side job while the kids were in school or the younger two were napping or at preschool, but thought it might be hard to find something that would allow me to work from home and on my schedule. I don't know if this person ever mentioned this to Kelly, but I soon found myself helping with the business. What started with just organizing and completing payroll for the two employees at the time to learning and taking over the business software, Kelly came to my rescue as much as I did to hers.

I'm now responsible for handling all administrative tasks, including scheduling, payroll, addressing client queries, managing their accounts, and the administration component to launch and support new programs. I'm a catch-all and do what I can to support Kelly and the team.

As a participant in KBC for fifteen years, I've developed and grown personally and professionally. Although I may slip up occasionally, the positive impacts of working out have carried over into other areas of my life. These habits have spread to my children through healthy eating or staying active. I have unconsciously learned and applied these habits to other areas of my life and the people I care about. What started as a desire to get in shape has become much more than that, and I'm grateful for the positive changes.

I've heard people outside of KBC consider Kelly's Bootcamp a cult. It may seem overwhelming for some personalities to come in and see that everyone knows each other. However, regulars are aware of this and make an effort to welcome newcomers and make them feel at home.

My favorite mantra of Kelly's is "Get what you came for," because that sentiment was asked of me in a plank position at LifeTime many years ago. To that, I add, "But you never know what you're going to get." Because at KBC, it's about more than just a workout. Our goal is to constantly innovate and evolve, providing our clients with more than what they know they need and always keeping everything fresh and new.

Kelly's Take

Therese's story makes me laugh. She's right. I don't remember her coming to my class at LifeTime, but based on her experience, it sounds like she only went to one. I taught at several commercial gyms, and we never had a roster of our students, so learning the names was a challenge. When I started KBC, that was one of the things that I wanted to solve, and many remember the handcrafted name tags that categorized the crew into teams as a Saturday bootcamp staple. This also helped members get to know each other.

I was cautious about announcing my bootcamp to my students in a class at another gym. Word spread to my students, and several of my original bootcampers have taken my classes since before KBC was born. When I had started the Saturday program, I had no intention of adding weekday classes, but Olympus, one of the gyms I taught at several evenings a week, shut down without warning, and those members were displaced. I promised them I could continue to offer the classes that I taught there at the same time, in my outdoor location. This unexpected setback was an opportunity and a solution to a problem for some of my most loyal students.

I appreciate that the Saturday early morning bootcamp was convenient for busy parents with children in sports and activities. Since it was in the neighborhood, parents could come to the early class and still get their kids to the field, court, or gym by 9:00 a.m. By adding the weekday evening classes, some of my Saturday bootcampers could build upon the progress that they were making with a once-a-week program.

I promised convenience, affordability, and fun when I started the outdoor program. It checked those boxes for Therese and many others.

Sometimes, it's a good thing if you need to improve at handling the administrative side of a business (for a long time, I just had an envelope in the front seat of the van). My lack of organization attracted Therese because she likes to help and solve problems. Therese didn't require much guidance as she understood the business and the people involved. Her skills were a perfect match for what we needed. When she stepped up as a Winter Challenge leader, I saw a whole new creative side to her.

Being introverted did not stop her from being a tremendous leader and bringing the best out in others around her.

The book "Who Not How" by Benjamin Hardy and Dan Sullivan discusses that you don't need to know how to do everything. When your goals outgrow your skill set, you need the right who. Fortunately, my greatest strength is attracting talented, honest, and hardworking people. The fact that Therese loved the organization and administrative work, as well as the KBC Community, was another sign that I was on the right path and able to grow from just a one-girl van in a parking lot. You must pay attention when the universe has its hand on your back trying to guide you.

Therese is the driving force behind everything we do at KBC. I like to refer to her as the wheels on the bus; nothing moves without her. She is organized, detail-oriented, wise, intelligent, candid, and hardworking, and she truly cares about KBC, the team, and the community. She is also a dear friend and confidant. She has seen me at my worst, yet she always supports me and the mission of KBC. There is no chance that I would be able to operate and grow without her.

Therese mentioned the Winter Challenge during her interview. She and four other mothers, who barely knew each other, were grouped to form a team named Team Chloe (after one of the team member's pets who had passed away at the beginning of the challenge). Therese was the captain of the team. Nobody knew what to expect since it was the first Winter Challenge, but it's fair to say that nobody expected Team Chloe to win. The moms on this team were active members of the community and the kind of people who focused more on the needs of others than themselves. But when they came together, magic happened:

At the end of the winter challenge I host an awards ceremony at my house. This is what I said to all those attendance as I announced that Team Chloe had won. "You demonstrated two of my favorite mottos: "Work for what you want" and "Get what you came for." You were an inspiration to everyone. Your contest win made all the parameters I said make sense. I knew the team that worked the hardest would win. You are a diverse group of individuals who found strength in loss and life changes. While there might have been some speculation, the numbers don't lie. You deserve this win 100%."

Everything Is Figureoutable

Asking for help used to be my kryptonite, but it has become my superpower. I call it my superpower because asking for help within my business benefits everyone involved. It goes far beyond helping just me. It makes my business better for the participants. It empowers my team to become more confident and more capable. Despite that, I used to avoid asking for or accepting help. I used to think I should be able to do everything myself. But that has all changed.

This change didn't happen overnight. I began to see the positive impact on the people I allowed to step up and help within the KBC community. I realized that permitting people to use their gifts and talents to contribute builds a stronger community. My need for help and my ability to ask for it was strong during the 2020 global pandemic.

In early 2020, my fitness business was booming. We had a community of over 400 people participating in regular workouts, nutrition, health promotion programs, and challenges designed to enhance and improve all aspects of wellness. We were at the top of our game. Lives were changing for the better. New students were falling in love with becoming fit, the KBC team was strong and energized, and we celebrated incredible transformations and small wins daily.

Then, in March 2020, when the COVID-19 pandemic hit, all our opportunities for in-person services were taken away. We had to find ways to keep our members engaged and moving. I knew our services had become a lifeline to our community and were needed more than ever, but we lacked the infrastructure to deliver.

Technology had never been an area I excelled in. Like everyone else in 2020, my heart was spread thin, and my brain was filled with anxiety and worry. But I knew that I had to step up. This was a season to put aside all of my own self-care, personal rules, and protect-your-passion mantras. Instead, it was time to figure out how to keep my community happy and healthy during the most challenging times.

I had just finished reading the book "Everything is Figureoutable" by Marie Forleo. I related to the author's passion for many of what seemed like unconnected things and building a business from the ground up. Her story reminded me of my own. The book's title, which was Forleo's mother's advice to her, became the new words inside my head.

The book states, "The most powerful words in the universe are the words you say to yourself." I repeated the words "**Everything Is Figureoutable**" to myself and my community repeatedly during that time. The words became the most powerful mantra during that season. In a way, this overshadowed my regular mantras, like "Just Show Up" and "Stay in Your Lane." But, in another way, it intensified all of it. Phrases like "Everything Matters" and "Don't Be Afraid to Fail" had more power than ever before.

In the book, Marie Forleo says, "If it's important enough, I'll make time. If not, I'll make an excuse." I have learned so much from this quote and put it into action. I stopped talking about things I said I wanted to do because I would have done them if they were important enough. Instead, I focused my energy on what I was making time for. This was especially important during the pandemic as I was faced with recreating how we delivered our services.

The power of **Everything Is Figureoutable** is indescribable. I would feel blocked and exhausted, and the simple reference to this phrase became my lifeline. These words allowed me to ask for help in a way I would never have been willing to. I could focus and concentrate on finishing tasks and projects that were far beyond my skill set. And most importantly, I genuinely believed, and still do believe, that anything is possible. I can find a way to make it happen. I can figure it out. And asking for help was the most essential part of making it happen.

Everything Is Figureoutable became my new power. I still say these words anytime I can't figure out how to put something together, run a report, manage a class, or solve a problem that seems too big to tackle. Now, these words remind me of successes, the times that I didn't know what to do and figured it out. They bring to mind the help I got to keep all classes running and the hundreds of people prioritizing home workouts and virtual accountability programs.

Everything Is Figureoutable, but that doesn't mean I have to be able to figure it out on my own. Instead, much of the time, I need to find somebody else who can figure it out—or someone who can figure it out with me.

None of this is to say that the pandemic was not challenging for the business, myself, and my team. I didn't feel qualified to make the kind of decisions that had to be made regarding the pandemic. I'm a rule follower by nature, but some rules were conflicting, opinions were strong, and the stakes were high. I relied heavily on Candice, a medical professional within our community. I was grateful for her professionalism and advice.

During the COVID-19 pandemic, we experienced a significant loss of around 20% of our membership base. Members canceled or put their memberships on hold for various reasons stemming from the difficult circumstances of the pandemic. Some did not adapt well to the virtual training options we had to shift to and preferred to try home fitness alternatives like Peloton. For others, the mental and emotional toll of the pandemic made it extremely challenging to maintain an exercise routine amidst all the other stresses and disruptions they were dealing with in their daily lives. The loss of these members was difficult. However, we were proud that most people retained their membership. I think those who stayed noticed how hard we worked. We found a way to serve our clients by offering high-quality virtual workouts and programs at times that worked best for our community. We stayed connected to our members, communicating daily and asking what they needed. We even opened up our memberships to the entire family. We loved seeing family members participating on the camera, pets included.

We have always offered the highest quality of our work, and virtual classes were no different. If we were going to add live-streamed classes, they had to be great, not just OK. I bought a course online from a mentor, and I contacted other business owners in the industry. I just kept educating myself and asking for help.

In her book "You Are a Badass," Jen Sincero said, "The only failure is quitting. Everything else is just gathering information." I refused to quit. I even refused to cancel classes, events, or community traditions. I kept gathering information, asking for help, and empowering my team. We always figured out a way. We changed Wi-Fi providers and called in a sound company. We were relentless in making this thing work. Keep in mind that I still don't have a good grasp of technology. I just found people who did.

We built a system inside Inergy (our indoor studio) that allowed each instructor to enter the building alone, teach a live class to our community in their homes, and save that workout to build what would become our video library.

When we were permitted to have a limited number of people inside the studio, our instructors simultaneously taught those in the studio and those who were live-streaming at home. We continued to experience and resolve tech issues. We all persisted in developing our teaching skills in new ways that benefited at-home participants and in-studio participants.

We maintained our offerings through Zoom and livestream because we wanted our members to continue taking the classes they loved with the instructors to whom they felt connected.

We sent most of our fitness equipment home with our members at no charge. We loaned out everything from hand weights to rowers to step benches. We gifted bender balls and workout bands. These things were used from home to make the virtual workouts more effective. But more importantly, it was the most authentic way to mimic the feel of our studio and parking lot workouts.

Instead of taking things away, we continued to give more. The entire team stepped up in every way possible. We became comfortable in front of the camera and resilient when faced with tech issues. We partnered with Fitgrid for technology, Myzone for heart rate monitoring, and even Michelob Ultra. They started a campaign with local fitness companies. I guess it takes a pandemic for a fitness business to partner with a beer company.

We continued all of our traditions and over-delivered in so many ways. We dropped off gift boxes on the porches of many of our members. We hosted a virtual Winter Challenge. We hand-delivered and mailed goal-setting journals to our clients. As soon as we could, we started bringing small groups of our clients back together at our outdoor lot and our studio, all while continuing to offer options to work out at home.

My biggest lesson from the pandemic is that people need people. People will achieve more when helping others than they will ever achieve for themselves. When we were all forced to isolate, connection through movement became powerful. Exercise choice and program design mattered less, and the laughs and virtual hugs became the most significant.

What Are We Training For? is a saying I might shout out while leading a workout. While it can be very literal, like training for a triathlon, it also has a deeper meaning. We're all training for something, even if we don't know what that something is. During the pandemic, I realized the KBC Dream Team had been training for this moment for years.

Our programming has always been organic, based on the community's current needs. We excel at being responsive and flexible with our offerings. From the very beginning, I've always added and modified programming because there was a direct need.

The KBC team has always been empowered to teach and train authentically. They've been encouraged to offer classes and programming that follow their own interests and expertise. As a result, each team member has consistently over-delivered in serving our community.

As a leader, I was extremely proud of how the team stepped up, putting their own insecurities aside, to empower our community to stay healthy and connected. We were all on a mission together, and that was powerful.

When I refer to "the KBC team" during the pandemic, I'm referring to people beyond our paid team. A faithful member, Trung, stepped up in a big way and became our volunteer tech support. He came in with a lot of knowledge and continued to learn along the way. He was at the studio countless hours serving as tech support for the entire team.

Today, in 2024, we still utilize the system we implemented in 2020. This was what we had been training for. This was the moment that answered the question **What Are We Training For?** As a community and team, we used everything we knew to make it through the pandemic and come out stronger on the other side.

Everything Is Figureoutable:

Borrowed from Marie Forleo. Approach everything you do with a can-do attitude. Anything is possible and can be figured out. You don't have to do it alone, though. Often, "figuring it out" means asking for and receiving help.

What Are We Training For?

This question can be quite literal. Are you training for a triathlon? Or maybe trying to lose weight? But the deeper meaning is this. We're all going to face adversity. Being physically and mentally strong will allow us to overcome.

Kristen's Story

I began as a participant in an outdoor Saturday bootcamp in 2014, shortly after having my first baby. It didn't last long because I became pregnant with my second in the fall, and I thought, "I can't work out; I'm pregnant." I started back in 2015, doing outdoor bootcamp, eventually adding some weekday classes. I liked the community and that Kelly knew my name, and whenever I would take one of her classes, it was like I always came away with something.

Making friends like Erica (who was also an instructor with KBC) and having workout buddies is what really kept me going. Now, the story of how I became an instructor is funny. I was at Kelly's class at Inergy one morning and asked for a band-aid because my shoes were rubbing my feet weirdly. And so we're in the bathroom, and she's getting me a band-aid, and she says, "Have you ever thought about becoming an instructor?" Surprised, I hadn't considered it before, despite my love for fitness. The idea kind of lingered throughout the rest of the class.

I don't know. I guess I could be an instructor. I don't love talking in front of people, but I really like fitness. I was a stay-at-home mom. I was like, maybe this would be fun. I just said yes.

By the time I finished my training and was ready to teach my first class, it was June 2020. Because of the pandemic, it was outside, we could only have ten participants, and we had to be separated. Despite the newness and the restrictions, I just loved teaching fitness classes.

It was just such an organic way of becoming an instructor. I didn't approach Kelly. She approached me. And now I can't imagine not teaching classes. I'm very passionate about it, and I've learned so much over the years. It's been almost four years.

Kelly had so much confidence in me that I started believing I could be a great instructor. Later on, she tells me, "I just have this knack for finding good people. I spot talent." After I gained some experience teaching, she hit me with, "See, I was right."

I think the transition from participant to instructor was smooth because the people at KBC truly support one another, and their generosity and kindness align with how I want to live my life. I enjoy volunteering and giving back, and that sense of community resonates with me.

Kelly often emphasizes the question, "What's your purpose for being here?" For me, it's about providing my kids with a positive example of being active since I didn't have that role model growing up.

I kept teaching during my third pregnancy and initiated a Mom & Me Baby program after my son's birth. Kelly's unique quality is her belief in people—she encouraged me to start a Mommy & Me class a couple of years ago, assuring me it would be great. It was a fantastic experience for the other moms and me. She believes in individuals and provides freedom in structuring classes, making it a cool and enjoyable experience.

Kelly's Take

The band-aid incident was a long-awaited one. Kristen, despite being a young mom, consistently prioritized fitness, standing out as a strong team player and leader in Saturday bootcamp for years. She was constantly receiving shout-outs for personal improvements, not just for her athleticism and energy but mainly for her can-do attitude.

Kristen's positivity and infectious energy make her a joy to be around. I knew our members would be attracted to her energy, and she was also someone with whom I knew the current team and I could easily work.

The fact that she said yes to taking on a role that she never considered herself for did not surprise me because I could see her confidence and yes-you-can attitude for five years as a student. Becoming an instructor through the pandemic is not something I think many people could have done. She only had a few in-person experiences before she started having to teach to a camera in an empty studio. I vividly recall showing her the complex studio setup and a detailed to-do list. She simply said, "I'll figure it out."

Kristen's innate desire to create a welcoming and comfortable environment was evident from the start. Unlike many new instructors, she focused on her students rather than worrying about doing everything perfectly. During the pandemic, KBC aimed to nurture and care for our students, and Kristen's ability to prioritize their well-being naturally stood out. It remains her superpower to this day.

So much of Kristen's story is part of what I want the reader of this book to take away. If it's something that stirs some excitement in you, just say yes! Don't overthink it.

Kristen could have used the pandemic as an excuse to delay her career as a fitness professional, but instead, she said, "I'll figure it out." This gave her a foundational connection with our members and is one reason she is adored by so many today.

Start. You'll never be fully ready. Show up with the attitude that you'll figure it out, focusing on making your students feel welcome and successful, creating the experience you want them to have after finishing a workout with you.

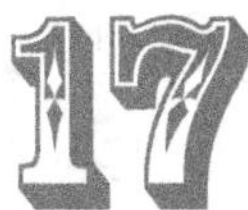

This Workout Belongs to You

During the pandemic, I started thinking specifically about coaching men and bringing them together. The KBC community has always been diverse in many ways, including offering our programs to men and women. However, I started noticing during the pandemic that women seemed to find a way to stay connected, but men seemed to be more isolated. Around the time I started thinking about what our community could specifically offer to men, two things happened.

First, I listened to a podcast about a program designed to help men with their health and fitness. It was aligned with my own goals, but the program was likely cost prohibitive for a lot of men. The voice inside my head said "Men need this right now. I can do this, make it more affordable, and make it more fun."

Second, I became aware of some friends I'd known growing up "gifting their birthdays" to their son, Alex. Alex Duncan, born with many physical challenges, including blindness, had outlived all the predictions made by doctors throughout his life. Now a twenty-five-year-old, Alex was diagnosed with testicular cancer. His parents posted on social media that they would forgo their own birthdays and friends should send cards and messages to Alex instead. A local news channel shared Alex's story of his lifelong fight, his parents' viral message, and strangers all over the country sending cards.

I was incredibly moved by Alex's parents' gesture and the outpouring of support that resulted. I thought to myself, "if strangers can send birthday cards to Alex in his final months, I can do my part too." Along with a birthday card, I decided to send a monetary gift. Alex wanted to use that gift to help others by "paying it forward." Shortly after, Alex and his parents started The Alex G. Duncan Foundation to help other men battling testicular cancer.

Many of the mantras and lessons in this book began to take shape. I decided to listen to the whispers and to **Just Start**. The next step in KBC's **Slow Organic Growth** was called Dude Camp. My vision of starting a program for guys to connect, relieve stress, and add a few extra workouts was coming to life.

When this vision became connected to Alex, it became powerful. **It's Got to Mean Something to You**. And now it did. We sent 100% of the proceeds from the inaugural session to the Alex G. Duncan Foundation.

Following my own mantra, **Don't Be Afraid to Fail**, I started very small. Our studio space was used most evenings and still limited because of COVID-19 restrictions. So I started the workouts in the garage of my house. The dudes began to connect with each other during workouts, through a group text chain, and in other areas of life. I believe that helping these men care for themselves creates a **Ripple Effect**. If we take care of the men in our community, it will impact the lives of many. **Creating Impact Starts with One Person**. The men of Dude Camp are leaders, fathers, and coaches. They often carry the weight of the world on their shoulders.

Dude Camp workouts are just once per week. While many of the dudes workout other times during the week, some can only make time for this one workout. Like all of us, several of the men in the group have physical issues—knees, hips, back. I emphasize that they should **Focus on What You Can Do**. I encourage them to come when they can and move in a way that honors their bodies.

People Will Always Do More for Other People Than They Will Do for Themselves. Dude Camp is proof of this statement. Created specifically for men who like the idea of being on a team, Dude Camp is full of challenges that lead to accountability and encouragement. Being a member of a team and raising money for a cause, for a cause, has led to the dudes participating regularly and in many situations taking their fitness to the next level.

The creation of Dude Camp has been tremendously rewarding to me personally. I know that I've made a difference in the lives of the men who participate while also benefiting a cause that means something to all of us. I also know that without all the other steps I've taken to create and build the KBC community, I would not have been in a position to start Dude Camp. It was an outcome I didn't imagine when I led that first Black Friday Bootcamp. But I know that one thing led to another, and I arrived exactly where I was supposed to be.

Alex passed on April 14, 2021, but his legacy lives on through his foundation. Shortly after Alex passed away, I sent this message to the dudes: Alex Duncan never stopped fighting, learning, and growing, and despite battles and obstacles since birth, he had a power and presence about him that inspired others. **It's Never Just a Workout**.

This Workout Belongs to You. It's your turn to start. You have everything you need to pursue your goals. Whatever it is you want to do, it's time to do it. Just start. You're likely to create impact, starting with just one person.

This Workout Belongs to You:

You're in charge of your own actions and impact. This applies literally to a physical workout. A good instructor can only do so much for you. Ultimately, you have to decide to give it your all. Figuratively, it can apply to so many other aspects of life.

Bob's story

I started KBC about a year ago when I was fifty-three. A friend I used to run with about ten years ago had joined KBC a few years prior. I had stopped running and wasn't looking for anything then. I play a lot of golf, and I walk when I play golf. I easily walk seven or eight miles three days a week, but my doctor told me that wasn't enough. I have realized that, especially as you get older, you need to continue to build your muscle mass. I've watched people around me, family members, and people I really care about not doing well as they get old. My doctor said "Listen, Bob, dying is easy. It's living like an invalid that's hard." That led me back to my old running buddy, Ted. He suggested giving KBC a try.

I knew it was going to be a good fit right away. I went to Kelly's Dude Camp class. It's a bunch of like-minded guys. It reminds me of gym class. Looking around, you can tell these guys excelled in gym. It's all really good guys who love it and want to be there. Every once in a while, she'll even let us play some dodgeball or something. A fifty-four-year-old guy who gets to play dodgeball, right? What's better than that? So I went to a Dude Camp on a Sunday and fell in love with it immediately because it was just something for me. It was intense.

Kelly's intense, and I love that about her. She's not going to let you slack in the class.

I want to grow old, as healthy and strong as possible. I still have a long road ahead, and I want to enjoy it. I think you see people who didn't take care of themselves, and you see the ailments they're dealing with and things that are entirely preventable through diet and exercise.

Kelly's Take

Bob is one of my favorite students (you'll hear me say that a lot because it's true). Bob played football in college. I could tell that he was an athlete before he ever told me. He's got the size of a collegiate football player for one. But it's so much more than that. It's the way he moves, the positive attitude he brings when he walks in the door, the way he encourages others in class, and his coachability. It's so fun to train him. Bob still plays a lot of golf, has added strength and conditioning workouts, and has improved his diet based on that conversation with his doctor. Today, he has body fat under 20% and is nearly back to his college playing shape at fifty-four!

Control the Controllables

I firmly believe I control my thoughts, focus, effort, commitment, and attitude. Concentrating on managing these aspects of my life makes me feel more confident and productive in my daily activities.

As the renowned motivational speaker Wayne Dyer once said, "We may not always have control over what happens around us, but we can always control our reactions to it."

This particular mantra has been a constant in my life since I was a child and is the most significant lesson I want to share in this book and with the people that I coach. There will always be hard things in your life that you cannot change, and focusing on what you can do is the secret sauce to not being defeated.

As you read through the stories of some of my most successful students, you will see how controlling physical health and giving back are through lines in their stories.

Here are some examples of how I **Control the Controllables** in my own life. The controllables are just what they sound like. They're the aspects of your life that you can assert some control over.

Helping Others. When my cousin Brett was battling leukemia, I felt utterly powerless against the disease. I was young, and so much of the conversations around his treatment were difficult to understand. But I was home from college for the summer and stepped up to live with and help care for his little sisters, giving them love and stability when everything else seemed uncertain.

During the pandemic, I couldn't help those fighting for their lives against a disease that was unpredictable and deadly. But I could remind my community that daily movement, even done in their living room, would better equip them to stay positive and keep them connected to their community.

Positive Thoughts. I have developed the ability to redirect my thoughts when they veer in a negative direction. Through practice and determination, I've become skilled at maintaining an upbeat and optimistic mindset most of the time. I've learned that by actively looking for the silver lining, I can cultivate a more positive outlook on life.

Exercise and Anxiety. I make no apologies for loving to exercise, but the movement is more than just a healthy activity I enjoy. Exercise is how I control my anxiety.

It's a bit of a running joke among my friends that they don't invite me for coffee or lunch because I have difficulty sitting and relaxing when I believe there's work to be done. I thrive on productivity, and remembering that there are times when slowing down and recharging is essential was, and still can be, very challenging for me.

I even had to quit a mastermind group that I loved for a period of time because I struggled to sit on the calls without feeling anxious. I'm not entirely sure why I experience this anxiety, but I do know that from a young age, I've used sports, exercise, or movement to help manage my restlessness, stress, and nervous energy.

I'm still a work in progress, but I've come a long way. I'm so passionate about helping people add consistent exercise into their routines because I know it can be just as beneficial for our mental health as it is for our physical well-being.

Physical activity is a natural stress reliever, releasing endorphins that elevate mood and reduce stress. The coping mechanisms developed during challenging workouts can be applied to navigate stress in everyday life. Whether facing a tight deadline at work or handling personal challenges, people who have found confidence through exercise often exhibit improved stress management skills.

The journey to finding confidence through physical activity is a powerful process. As we see what we can do, set and reach our goals, and build discipline, the confidence we gain with exercise spreads to other parts of our lives. When we take a comprehensive approach to well-being, where physical and mental health are connected, we can become more confident and satisfied with our lives.

Let's explore the basics of this concept: **Control the Controllable**. A big part of controlling the controllables is to recognize the many things you cannot control. Everyone's situations are different, but there are a few common things most of us can control. We can care for our physical health, practice gratitude, surround ourselves with positivity, and talk kindly to ourselves.

Let's visit each of these controllables in more detail.

Take Care of Your Physical Health

Exercise, good nutrition, and sleep are basic staples in my life. I discovered that I could easily control these things when I was very young. Over the years, when I've had success in these areas, I've also found success in other areas of my life. I've gained confidence to reach for and achieve other goals by tending to these basics.

Exercise doesn't have to be complicated. Any activity that moves your body works. The secret is to start with something small that you can build on. Once you succeed with that one thing, ask yourself what else you can do. Taking on too much at once can be overwhelming and rarely leads to consistent success. By starting small, you'll likely gain confidence and feel powerful by building on your personal success. Recognize your success and reward yourself with the next step. Keep the energy positive; don't get down on yourself for what you didn't do.

Having a support system that wants the best for you makes the journey more fun and likely to continue. You can find that support system in so many different ways. Joining a local fitness community can be one way to find that support system. But there are also online communities, running clubs, tennis leagues, and so much more.

The most important thing when making movement a regular part of your life is to find an activity you enjoy. You're much more likely to stick with it. Don't waste your time and energy with fad programs or crazy workouts. When a potential client inquires about a workout program, my first question is whether they enjoy it. My follow-up assessment is the potential for long-term commitment and growth. If the response to either of these is negative, I advise against the program and consider it a waste of their time. A good workout program is one you'll stick with. We only continue long term with things we enjoy.

The link between physical activity and overall confidence is a well-established phenomenon. Physical activity is not just about building muscle or shedding calories. It can be a powerful catalyst for building confidence that transcends beyond the gym or workout space.

Here are some ways physical activity can help foster confidence:

Setting and Achieving Goals

Engaging in regular physical activity often involves setting fitness goals. This might be running a certain distance, lifting a specific weight, or mastering a challenging yoga pose. As people experience their own progress and accomplishments in exercise, it instills a sense of achievement. This newfound ability to set and achieve goals in the physical domain can translate seamlessly to setting and accomplishing personal and professional goals.

Improved Self-Image

Regular exercise contributes to both physical well-being and a positive self-image. As people notice positive changes in their bodies, they often develop a more accepting and appreciative attitude toward themselves. This enhanced self-perception can have a ripple effect on overall self-confidence, influencing how people perceive and present themselves in various life situations.

Enhanced Social Confidence

Participating in group fitness classes, team sports, or even solo workouts in a public setting provides opportunities for social interaction. The camaraderie fosters social confidence. People who are initially reserved or shy often find their social skills improving as they connect with others who share similar fitness goals. This expanded social confidence extends beyond the gym, positively impacting interactions in various social settings.

Discipline and Consistency

Building a regular exercise routine requires discipline and consistency. This commitment to physical well-being instills valuable life skills in other areas. People who learn to prioritize and dedicate time to their health often find themselves better equipped to manage their time and commitments in other aspects of life. The discipline cultivated through physical activity becomes a foundation for success in diverse endeavors.

Nutrition and movement go hand in hand. Good food fuels your body. Eating whole foods that you enjoy and nourish your body will go a long way. You don't have to be perfect with this. Start making small changes that become part of who you are. Anyone can be perfect for a short time, but it won't move the needle in your overall health unless it's something you keep doing. For example, exercising and eating well don't have to be complicated. Find foods you enjoy that also nourish your body. Eat those foods most of the time but accept that you'll also eat other foods sometimes.

The third part of caring for your physical health might be the most critical. Sleep is so important. Making sleep a priority will help with every aspect of your life.

According to the Sleep Foundation, adults need seven or more hours of sleep every night. A study from 2024 concluded that more than one-third of adults get less than the seven-hour recommendation on average. Further, the study showed a link between using blue light-emitting devices before bed and the time it takes to fall asleep. Perhaps one small step you can take to ensure adequate sleep is to reduce screen time before bed.

Through my involvement in the Todd Durkin Mastermind, I've adopted the practice of following **Personal Rules**. Developing a completely personalized set of rules to follow is empowering. It gives me the authority to decide what I can and cannot control. My list of rules focuses on the positive things I can do every day to be healthier and happier.

I encourage you to develop your own personal rules. While everyone's rules should be customized, seeing my list as an example might be helpful.

Keep in mind that the goal is not perfection. As you might recall from a previous chapter, **Perfect Isn't There**. Personal rules are in place to remind us of what we're working toward. The goal is to follow the rules most of the time. I'm constantly revisiting, modifying, and reinstating these rules as my life ebbs and flows.

Kelly's Personal Rules

1. **Family of six at the table at least twice a week.** It's crucial to gather my family of six around the table as much as possible. (My older kids are away at college, so this is a summertime rule to be applied when everyone is again under the same roof.)

2. **Be mindful when in the presence of others.** Care and listen to others.

3. **Go to bed by 9:45 p.m.** Sunday through Friday. Morning bootcamp comes early!

4. **Avoid caffeine after 1:00 p.m.**

5. **Restrict alcohol to two days per week.** I do make exceptions to this for vacations and other special occasions.

6. **Vegetables and high-quality protein sources** at every meal and at least one snack.

7. **Minimum of 100 ounces of water per day.**

8. **Eat food only when sitting down.**

9. **Seventy percent of the time, eat food in its most natural form.** I recently changed this from 90% of the time. Seventy

percent seemed more reasonable. Therefore, I can stay more consistent on this one now.

10. **Chew slowly.** I'm always a work in progress. This is hardest when I come home hungry after teaching evening classes.

11. **Listen to, respect, and show gratitude toward my body.**

12. **Work out every day.** Walking counts.

13. **Channel my energy to the people who need it the most.**

14. **If I think something positive about somebody I care about, tell them.**

15. **Motivate, inspire, and create an impact in the lives of the KBC community.** This includes the KBC team.

16. **Allow for friend time and connections** with those who have positive energy.

17. **Protect my passion as a fitness professional.** Be guided by that passion.

18. **Therapeutic massage at least once per month**—more often when I can.

19. **Create my daily list and show myself grace if I don't get through it.**

Practice Gratitude

Another aspect we can control is how we approach the ups and downs of life. No matter what we're faced with, we can practice gratitude. I know this isn't the first time you've heard this, but there's a reason gratitude is so often talked about. It works.

If I'm mad I didn't get the number of things I set out to complete, I try to focus on what I did accomplish and that the extra time it took was worth it because I learned something or got to have a personal connection with someone.

Another practice I learned from the Todd Durkin Mastermind is **WLAGs** (wins, losses, a-has, and goals). Here's how it works. Simply list your wins during a specific period (the week, the month, the year). Write down everything that went well in your personal and professional life.

Next, list your losses. These are the things that didn't go so well— your disappointments.

Next, a-has. After listing your wins and losses, you'll no doubt think of several things you learned. Something that happened that made you say "a-ha."

And, last, goals. List some specific goals you have going forward.

The order matters. Listing wins first helps us practice gratitude. By recognizing all the things that went well, your frame of mind is grateful even as you move on to acknowledge your losses. Leaving goals to the end allows you to consider where you've been before planning where to go.

By writing my wins consistently, I've realized what I'm most grateful for: time spent with people I care about, having significance in the lives of others, and getting things done that are important to my mission as a mom, wife, business owner, and community member.

Surround Yourself with Positivity

Surrounding yourself with people who lift you up with inspiring messages is essential. In my younger years, it was friends, coaches, and bosses. As I've gotten older, in addition to surrounding myself with positive people, I also intentionally read and listen to messages about self-development from people who have found success in both career and life.

Changing the voice inside your head can happen by reading and listening to the right books, articles, and social media. Listening to educational and thought-provoking podcasts and webinars is inspiring. Surrounding yourself with growth-minded people who want the best for themselves and everyone around them is so important. Most importantly, you have to believe it's possible. You have to believe you can guide the voice in your head toward positivity.

In doing all of this, you can learn to **Talk Nicely to Yourself**. Think of how you would speak to a beloved friend. That's the same tone you should use with yourself. Showing yourself grace is one of the most important ways to surround yourself with positivity.

Practice Self-Care

Another thing that most of us can control is taking care of ourselves. Self-care is huge for me and something I used to be embarrassed about. I have always been far less concerned about material things and more interested in experiences that relieve stress and rejuvenate. Regular deep tissue massage, cranial sacral work, and relaxing facials are good for my mind and spirit. Even the anticipation of planning these services serves as a reset and release. Then, while I'm there, I can fully check out and relax.

Overcoming the guilt of spending time and money on self-care has been a process for me. Now, I can justify the time and money because every important role I have in life involves being lit up for other people. If I invest in myself, I'll be better equipped and have a longer career helping others.

Now it's your turn to **Control the Controllables**. You can start slowly and simply. Control what you can. Take care of your physical health. Take time to be grateful for what you do have and what you have already done. Make an effort to surround yourself with all things positive. Practice self-care.

Then, look at your circumstances and determine if are other controllables specific to your situation. Remember to also recognize the things you cannot control.

Control the Controllables

Recognize that there are certain aspects of your life that you cannot control. Then, focus on the aspects that you can control. We all have our unique circumstances, but some common controllables are physical health, gratitude, positivity, and self-care.

Personal Rules

A personalized set of rules that we aim to stick to most of the time. Following the rules should lead to health and happiness.

WLAGs

A practice of listing wins, losses, a-has, and goals from a designated period of time. The order matters. Listing wins first creates a feeling of gratitude through the rest of the practice.

> ## Talk Nicely to Yourself
>
> Think of how you would speak to a beloved friend. That's the same tone you should use with yourself.

Gretchen's Story

I started going to KBC in the summer of 2015 when Kelly was offering an end of summer promotion for a free August. I had been stalking them for two years, maybe three. During that time, I had a newborn and a two-year-old, and whenever I drove by, I would see people working out in the parking lot next to Harris Teeter at all hours of the day. I would drive by and think to myself, "This is insane. I'm not doing that. That's crazy."

No matter what I did on my own, I could not stick with it. I had what I lovingly called my box of fitness toys and videos, but nothing worked. I must have signed up for an email list at some point, and when I saw the promotion to try it, I sent a plea out to two of my girlfriends who were also in my neighborhood with kids of similar ages. We had all been lamenting about our new mom bodies and what we would do. And I was like, "I want to do this, but I know I won't do it if you don't do it with me; it'll be another thing that I quit in a month. Will you do it?" One of them said yes, and she is still a member. I just worked out with her at 5:15 a.m.

We both started with Saturday bootcamp. It was easy to stick with because it was fun. My friend was a teacher, and I had an office job, but within a couple of months, we picked up one or two other weeknight classes. Our husbands were excited that we were doing this; they cared for the kids and made dinner on the nights we went to class. Going to the parking lot to work out for an hour became this vacation, like a happy place where I got to meet up with a friend and forget all this stuff at home. My love for the bootcamp went from liking it to loving it and then needing it. I immediately noticed a positive change in both how I felt and looked.

Saturday bootcamps included many assessments so that you could measure yourself. I liked that you could track your improvement, whether a timed mile or not getting out of breath the first two minutes of the class. How many pushups can you do in a minute? How many sit-ups can you do in a minute? You could see, oh my God, I am getting stronger. I am getting faster.

That's important because that is the theme of my relationship with Kelly's Bootcamp. It became less about what I looked like and more about what I could do. And even that started to progress from not only what I can do physically but what I can do for myself, my life, and my mentality. It's what Kelly did, using my body to train my mind; you can do this! You didn't think you could do this, but now you can do it if you keep applying this to every aspect of your life. What else could you do?

The three things that Kelly says that speak to me are "two claps," "Easy doesn't make you better," and "Just show up." It's always about taking action.

Whenever I encounter something challenging, and it feels overwhelming, I remind myself that I have surprised myself in the past. I have achieved things that I didn't think were possible, such as doing a significant number of pushups or running a seven-minute mile. It's all about training the mind and body to work together.

I have a list of things I once thought were too difficult, but I now do them easily. Working with Kelly has taught me that growth and strength come from discomfort. Her coaching has taught me valuable life lessons that extend beyond just fitness. My experience with Kelly and my progress have become an example for any other area of my life that feels stagnant or too hard.

Kelly has a motto that says, "Change equals change." The idea behind this is change is necessary to grow on any level. Something has to be different if we want to be different. I have made significant progress in my fitness assessments, but KBC changes the schedule every season. As a result, I work with new instructors or try out new classes. These changes have benefited me because I have learned that even a small adjustment to an exercise can make it more challenging and help me become stronger. Sometimes, I change my life without knowing what I need, hoping it will lead me to something new and beneficial. This is a way to reframe life: Expect discomfort with change and be excited about the opportunities it can bring.

In my second year at KBC, Kelly made a call in one of her weekly emails about the Winter Challenge. I didn't know the Winter Challenge, but she sought challenge leaders. And the way she described it, it was a lot about service, and she's just looking for someone to help people. And I read it as, oh my gosh, anything I can do to give back to this community that has changed my life this last year and a half, yes, I'm all in. Cool, let's do it. I had no idea what I was getting into. Fast forward seven years, and I have been a captain six times. The teams have been anywhere from thirteen to twenty-two people. Being a challenge leader is the closest I feel I can be to getting inside Kelly's head, where you are just motivated by seeing people get better and having a level of certainty about what people can do even when they don't believe it.

I also love that despite the competition, it brings out the best in people because they are committed to showing up for their team. I'm doing more in these two months because I'm part of this team, and I don't want to let these people down.

It's inspiring to feel that you matter and see your contributions to a team and what you're capable of when you do not know what you can and can't do. Instead, it's this unparalleled type of optimism and grit—like, yeah, team, we got this, and we did this, the high fives, the celebrations, and the parties. So that's been another just a-ha. If you don't think you can do something, find an external person to tie it to, and then the action becomes more significant than you. That's the power of the community.

Kelly's Take

I have learned so much from Gretchen in the past ten years. She showed up so strong and determined that it was hard to believe she watched us from afar, lacking confidence for so long before starting. So how do you go from that's crazy, I would never do that to I love it, I need it? You never will unless you start. Gretchen thinks a lot; she gets inside her head, which can be powerful but also limiting.

The investment was minimal, but the reward was high, and that decision to put herself out there started with her own two-clap moment before we even met. I always think it's never about price when it comes to starting, but her stories and many others I have heard from my members have proven me wrong. It's about eliminating barriers, and I understand that some people don't want to invest in themselves until they believe they are committed. Gretchen didn't think she would stick with KBC when she started, but she was smart enough to address her concerns by gaining the support of friends and connecting to her *why* of losing the baby weight and feeling like herself again when she started.

I ran bootcamps and outdoor classes for six years before Gretchen joined. Over the years, I have witnessed many remarkable transformations in the fitness community and realized the importance of inviting more people to join us. This prompted us to offer a free month before the start of our fall program, as we wanted to reach out to those who may benefit from our community, even if they were unaware of it. My motivation to attract more people stems from my belief that physical fitness can act as a catalyst for achieving one's goals in other aspects of life. Gretchen is an incredible example of this.

Gretchen mentions some of the mantras I tell my students to help them spring into action. The one she does not say, but I hear as she describes her journey into motherhood, is control the controllables. Listening to people's stories is one of the distinct honors I get as a coach. Sometimes, it's the story that they tell themselves, and other times, it's really what has happened to them. In Gretchen's case, it happened: She lost her identity and felt like if she could fit into her old clothes, she would get it back. By taking action, she immediately felt better and looked better. It allowed her to do other things. I know this story will resonate with other moms, and I'm grateful Gretchen shared it so openly and honestly.

I wanted to address a common misconception about people who work out. When we see someone incredibly fit and consistent with exercise, we often assume they've always been that way and that it comes easily to them. However, this is only sometimes true. In Gretchen's case, she struggled with sticking to a program. She had all the tools but needed more structure and motivation. She started with a low commitment a few times a week and got hooked on improving herself. It wasn't about being the best but rather about getting better. During the early years of bootcamp, I conducted many assessments, not because the numbers mattered but because I wanted to provide my students with proof that they were improving. Coaching personal improvement has proven to be a highly effective motivator for them to keep going, and it worked for Gretchen and countless others. We are constantly assessing progress today, but we don't always have to count reps to see it.

After achieving something new, we ask ourselves, "What else can I do?" This is what we call building upon our success. Gretchen signing up to be a Winter Challenge leader was most certainly an opportunity for her to give back to a program that had given so much to her, but it was also an example of how when you master a new skill and find success, you desire to teach and empower others to do the same.

Gretchen has a remarkable ability to lead a team, which is her superpower. She draws her strength from her intelligence, confidence, love, and understanding of people. During the Winter Challenge for several years, it didn't matter who I assigned to her team; they always ended up being a success story. KBC's team members' experience, track record, age, ethnicity, gender, or level of athleticism were insignificant. Once they became a part of Gretchen's team, they consistently achieved extraordinary results, formed strong bonds, and had an experience beyond physical health and fitness.

In 2023, the Challenge team was exceptionally strong. Gretchen led a diverse team of women, including some Winter Challenge rookies and others who had tried everything but had yet to achieve their desired results. The team's culture was to embrace difficult challenges and wear them as a badge of honor in the team's name. One of Gretchen's teammates was fighting for her life. This widow was battling leukemia and was trying to get into a life-saving clinical trial study for treatment but was denied due to her BMI. Gretchen and her team helped her achieve the necessary results to get into the study. The team was named the Legends that year and won the Challenge, but the real victory was its impact on the future.

Gretchen is a valuable KBC community member who is passionate about helping people achieve their health and fitness goals. She recognized the significance of the formula she created for her teammates and decided to earn her credentials to become a certified nutritionist. Since joining the team in 2023, Gretchen has conducted several workshops to assist our clients in customizing their macronutrient targets to maintain muscle and lose fat. She is an adept problem solver, an enthusiastic researcher, and a natural leader who enjoys teaching and supporting others.

I think Gretchen only considered becoming a nutrition coach once she worked with her 2023 team. She wanted to acquire the necessary credentials to expand her coaching skills and ensure that her advice was appropriate and within her scope of practice. Her ultimate goal was to leverage her successful track record as a winter contest leader to make a sustainable and realistic impact beyond the first few months of the year.

There are several valuable lessons we can learn from Gretchen's story. One particular quote from Robin Sharma's book, "The Greatness Guide," ties her story together beautifully: "What you give away comes back to you in a river." Although some may view the free month I gave away in 2015 as a poor business decision, my reason for doing it was to expand the positive impact we were having on people's lives and to extend that impact to even more individuals. This created a ripple effect where people began sharing what they learned, supported one another, and felt inspired to keep going. Helping and inspiring others is truly a rewarding experience that has no limits when it becomes part of your culture."

11 Reasons I Wanted to Write This Book

1. Synchronicities. I have found great happiness and fulfillment in my life, and I believe a big part of that comes from thinking that the synchronicities that occurred were reassurance that I was on the right path. It's not the things that happened but how my body and mind reacted. The best example I have of this is when I was at the BWI airport on January 11, the day my dad passed away. I felt the buzz of my cell phone on my lap, and when I picked it up and looked at the screen, I saw big letters: 11:11 Dad Calling. It was my younger brother Chris calling from my father's cell phone, but that was a powerful moment that stayed with me. After my father's death, countless significant communications would come through right at 1:11 or 11:11, the ones that would appear at times that felt meaningful. It wasn't something I talked about then; I just had this powerful feeling that comforted me.

2. Shared experiences. Over a year after my father's death, my stepmom Sheila was visiting with a few of my siblings, and we were sitting in the kitchen late into the evening, talking and telling stories. I looked at the wall oven clock and saw the digital red number 11:11.

I must have shuddered, and Sheila noticed and asked why. I explained that I felt like my father was with me when I saw a series of ones and described some of the meaningful examples. She went on to share some very specific examples of seeing the series of ones. My father was an electrician by trade, and she had unbelievable occurrences with the power in the house and the car, resulting in stopped clocks stopping with a series of ones on them. Of course, after this conversation, we all looked for the ones when we needed luck, guidance, or affirmation. It may sound crazy, but it meant something to us, which is all that mattered. We missed my dad. We wanted to feel and see him again, and this was our way of doing that.

3. Overcoming challenges. There are countless reasons that I shouldn't have started a company with so many moving parts. I'm very challenged with organization and don't have the skill set needed to run a business. I did it anyway, and almost on cue, the right people appeared to bridge the gap. In addition, I find it reassuring that technological advancement and the ability to use software and apps to solve many organizational aspects of running a fitness business have become accessible and user-friendly.

4. Symbolism. When I named my studio "Inergy," I liked that it played on the word "energy" because that made me think of my family's 100 years in business electrical contracting company (Schenectady Hardware & Electric). While designing the logo, I asked the designer to incorporate the three ones at the end of the word "Inergy." Some people might see it as a barbell, but I know that it represents 111.

5. Emotional epiphany. The night the Inergy sign went up, I saw it lit for the first time. It was so powerful that it moved me to one of the hardest and most intense cries that I had ever had in my life. It was at that moment that I knew my emotion was a sign that this was going to be a very special place and that powers had guided me outside of myself.

6. Unexpected support. I was very naive about all the permits required and inspections that would have to take place to open a brick-and-mortar fitness studio after a build-out. My mom was at the end of her life as I was opening Inergy, which compounded my struggle. Out of nowhere, a guy named Ryan appeared with the offer to oversee this aspect of the opening, charging very little and being an invaluable source of information and support.

7. Meaningful encounters. On the day of our soft opening, I hired a cleaning company to come in and clean the glass and mirrors. I was in the studio alone when I saw this very tan man with sunglasses who introduced himself as Larry. My father's name was Larry, he always wore sunglasses and had a tan, and he would have wanted that glass to shine.

8. Acts of kindness. I find it significant that Ginger gave me my first donation check to support my mission before I even knew her name or my mission. Later, she became the first person I allowed to help me and create an experience for our members that involved significant touchpoints and ways to connect beyond what I could at the time. I called her my bootcamp angel, always cheering for me and my mission. She started her own fitness business and impacted even more people. It's amazing how one person can help you believe that something is possible and the reciprocal effect that it can ultimately have. Ginger was a sign that more angels would come, and they did.

9. Collaboration. Like many people, I have said for years that I wanted to write a book. If asked why, I would say that I want to inspire others to believe in themselves. I want people to understand that the bad things in your life are good, and you have to begin and not overthink it or try to make it perfect.

Since I had been talking about it but never took action, I hired Emily. Emily and I met at a fitness conference. When she moved to Northern Virginia with her family, she was looking for a place to teach yoga, and we were reunited. She remembered me from the conference because we discussed naming my studio. Emily shared that she had a long career as a fitness professional and was also a fitness business owner of a brick-and-mortar studio at one point.

After she moved out of state, she emailed to share that she was starting a content writing business. I love supporting anyone starting a business. I could certainly use help with writing, and I was excited to work with Emily again. She finished an email campaign project for me, and I liked it. Just as important, I enjoyed working with her over Zoom. She was excited about her work, and I liked the energy she brought to our meetings. When I mentioned that I thought she could help me write a book, she devised a plan. The weekly meetings kept me on task and served as an emotional release for some of the heavier things I was writing about.

10. The power of people. Your relationships matter just as much as your workout routine and nutrition. My friends and family (many not blood-related) have lifted me up and given me purpose. Take, for instance, Chris Kerns, who I met when he was just sixteen and working at the café of the fitness center I managed (a job I didn't think I wanted). From that moment on, he became woven into the fabric of our family.

Over the years, through thick and thin, he has been a steadfast presence, offering unwavering support and love. When my father passed away unexpectedly, he was there. The same month, we stood by his side after the untimely death of his father. His role in our lives goes beyond friendship. He's a little brother to my husband and the cherished "crazy uncle" to all four of my children. His unwavering support and enthusiasm make him the biggest cheerleader for our family, demonstrating the profound impact of a relationship that began unexpectedly when he was just a teenager. Now, seeing him with his own family brings a joy I never could have anticipated—an extension of the love and connection we've shared over the years.

11. It's Got to Mean Something. Sometimes, I marvel at the seeming luck in my life. Why does my fitness business thrive while others struggle? Why does my passion for the industry never wane, even when burnout looms for so many? Why do I attract such a dedicated and talented team when finding such individuals is challenging across all fields? But then I realize it's not just luck—it's about doing work that genuinely means something to me. When you're passionate about what you do, success isn't merely chance. It's a natural outcome of dedication, purpose, and a genuine connection to your craft.

A Note from Emily

Working with Kelly on *Start Before You're Ready* has been life changing. My role was more than a collaborator. I was a student and a mentee of Kelly's. Through every conversation and every correspondence exchanged, I benefited from Kelly's wisdom. As I delved deeper into the information she wanted to share in the book, I was both inspired and challenged. I was inspired to put Kelly's wisdom and advice into action in my own life. And, I was challenged to help Kelly clarify her message and put in written form what she has been sharing for decades in her KBC community. I hope we got it right.

Kelly and I met years ago and I believe that the intertwining of our lives is not a coincidence. We were meant to work together on this book. We first crossed paths years ago at a fitness conference and have interacted with many of the same leaders in the fitness industry. When my family and I moved to Northern Virginia five years ago, our house was just a half mile from Inergy. During the two years we lived in the area, I taught yoga at KBC and Kelly and became friends. After moving back to Cincinnati, I decided to start a new career as a freelance writer. Kelly was one of my very first clients. I enjoyed working with her on a small project but was surprised at her next idea…help her write a book. I wasn't planning to take on projects of that size until I gained more experience.

Kelly assured me that I was the person she wanted to work with and that she believed in my abilities. She encouraged me, just as she has encouraged so many people in the KBC community. And now, I hope Kelly's words in this book have encouraged each of you to…*Start Before You're Ready*.

Acknowledgements

To **Emily Stapleton**: One of my favorite sayings is to enjoy the process, not just the outcome. Of course, I wanted this book to come to be, but even if it didn't, it still would've been worth it because of the insightful and powerful conversations that Emily and I had together. She is a trusted friend, confidant, coach, gifted writer, and listener. Writing this book was incredibly therapeutic, and I believe Emily was a big part of that. We did it.

I extend my heartfelt gratitude to the following individuals who generously provided candid interviews for "Start Before You're Ready":

Debbie Weigand, Amy Beyer, Heather Comerford, Meg Phillips, Margery Pratt, Jenny Greenfield, Jodi Austin, Kristen Kime, Gloria Monge, Rebecca Weaver, Mike O'Shea, Kathy Curtin, Kathy & Ted Moore, Julie McGee, Mohammad Khattak, Therese Barnes, Kristen Bridger, Bob Kehoe, and Gretchen Comey.

These inspiring individuals contributed to this book and are examples of starting before you're ready and embodying growth mindsets. Their stories and insights have enriched this work immeasurably.

To **ALL THOSE I ASKED FOR HELP**, Especially Nicole O'Shea, Jamie Lockwood, Amy Beyer, Christine Varanelli, Meg Philips, Debbie Weigand, Margery Pratt, Kristen Jackson, Traci Jersen, and Kris Gregory: Thank you for your insights and thoughtful contributions and for being my lifeline the many times I got stuck. Your support and feedback were invaluable.

To **Jen Newman**: Thank you for coming up with the name of the book while floating in Lake George. Whenever I see the cover, I'll think of you, Leah, and that sunny day.

To **Kelli Watson, Greg Justice**, and **Scriptor Publishing**: Thank you for creating a platform where wannabe authors can proudly hold a book in their hand.

To the **Todd Durkin Mastermind:** By surrounding myself with people I wanted to be more like, I could complete things I never thought I would.

To **Chandrika Sattiraju**: Thank you for being a game changer and showing up to photograph the lot and me.

www.ingramcontent.com/pod-product-compliance
Lightning Source LLC
Chambersburg PA
CBHW061033250726

48653CB00001B/82